Medicare

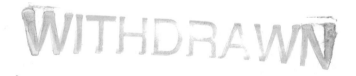

Marilyn Moon

Also of interest from the Urban Institute Press:

Health Policy and the Uninsured, edited by Catherine G. McLaughlin

Marilyn Moon

Medicare

A Policy Primer

THE URBAN INSTITUTE PRESS
Washington, D.C.

THE URBAN INSTITUTE PRESS
2100 M Street, N.W.
Washington, D.C. 20037

Library of Congress Cataloging-in-Publication Data

Moon, Marilyn.
  Medicare : a policy primer / by Marilyn Moon.
    p. ; cm.
  Includes bibliographical references and index.
  ISBN 0-87766-753-5 (pbk.: alk. paper)
  1. Medicare.   2. Medical policy--United States.   3. Health care reform--United
States.
  [DNLM: 1. Medicare--organization & administration. 2. Consumer Satisfaction--
United States. 3. Health Care Reform--United States. WT 31 M818ma 2006] I. Title.
  RA412.3.M658 2006
  368.4'2600973--dc22   2006005730

Printed in the United States of America

10 09 08 07 06 1 2 3 4 5

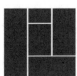 **THE URBAN INSTITUTE** is a nonprofit, nonpartisan policy research and educational organization established in Washington, D.C., in 1968. Its staff investigates the social, economic, and governance problems confronting the nation and evaluates the public and private means to alleviate them. The Institute disseminates its research findings through publications, its web site, the media, seminars, and forums.

Through work that ranges from broad conceptual studies to administrative and technical assistance, Institute researchers contribute to the stock of knowledge available to guide decisionmaking in the public interest.

Conclusions or opinions expressed in Institute publications are those of the authors and do not necessarily reflect the views of officers or trustees of the Institute, advisory groups, or any organizations that provide financial support to the Institute.

CONTENTS

INTRODUCTION

I have long been interested in the Medicare program, beginning many years ago when I examined the impact of government programs on the well-being of the elderly. While working at the Congressional Budget Office, I acquired a general knowledge of the program, and people at the Health Care Financing Administration and elsewhere provided help. But I found that many experts in the program knew, in enormous detail, only a portion of Medicare. My first book on Medicare, published in 1993, sought to offer a general view of the program from the viewpoint of beneficiaries. At that time, health care reform was being seriously debated, and I feared the book would be out of date as soon as it was released. Medicare was going to be folded into a larger program or at the least changed substantially.

But the health care reform failed, and instead of expansions in publicly financed health programs, it seemed substantial cutbacks and shifts away from social insurance would follow. In 1996, when I worked on the second edition of *Medicare Now and in the Future,* the program had just escaped major changes after a presidential veto. A scaled-down version of Medicare reforms passed in 1997 and led to major changes.

Medicare faced changes again in 2003, this time through the addition of a prescription drug benefit—the first major benefit expansion in Medicare's history. The new century also renewed efforts to rely on the private sector and on claims that Medicare is "unsustainable" and must be severely limited over time. This third volume on Medicare considers the impacts of the 2003 legislation, though the new law is yet to be fully implemented, much less understood. This volume is not a new edition, since so much change after nearly a decade demands a total reexamination of the program and the challenges it faces.

As Medicare turns 40, a larger midlife crisis seems to be underway. Much of the discussion on Medicare in the 1980s and 1990s focused on new ways to pay for care, changes that affected access to care, people's attitudes about the program, and the delivery system in general. Now the concern is whether the program will remain much the same or be transformed in more significant ways than has occurred through many years of budget tinkering and even major change.

My interest has always been on the beneficiary. Others have focused on the importance of the program to providers of health care services. Instead, I look more at the program's impact on those it serves and, in turn, the needs of the beneficiaries and how they place demands on Medicare. So I give relatively short shrift to the complicated payment systems that Medicare employs.

I confess to a bias to the belief that the vulnerability of the elderly and disabled populations, and the failure of the private sector to care adequately for them, has created an important role for a government program. To be sure, part of my conclusions are based on a desire to ensure a basic level of health care for them; but I also strongly believe that it is essential to examine the data and research on how best to meet these needs. For policy analysts, our work does not end with research on a topic. It is impossible to work in an area without developing conclusions about policy improvements. Most researchers also take on projects that interest or challenge them. Anyone who claims to be fully neutral before examining an issue is probably fooling themselves as well as their readers. That does not mean that valid research and analysis must be biased; indeed, I hope to look objectively at findings and respond when the evidence points in new and different directions. And while I have tried to keep my conclusions on the program to the last chapter, analysis and my choice of topics in earlier chapters obviously reflect my values.

The Urban Institute and the American Institutes for Research have both provided support for this effort. And I have drawn on my own research, which has been generously funded by the Commonwealth Fund and the Kaiser Family Foundation over the years. None of these institutions, of course, is responsible for the material contained herein. For that I take full responsibility.

I am grateful to many people who have influenced my thinking and encouraged my efforts over the years. A number of research colleagues have supported my efforts, including Cristina Boccuti, Stephanie Maxwell, and January Angeles who oversaw work by a raft of junior researchers. And those whose efforts made the numbers and charts contained in this volume possible include Misha Segal, Matt Storeygard, Krista Dowling, and Jenny Wong. Over the years of working in this area, I have benefited from debates and conversations with too many people to mention here, but I would be remiss without including a few. My colleagues at the Urban Institute, including John Holahan, Steve Zuckerman, Linda Blumberg, Tim Waidmann, and Korbin Liu were always willing to read and discuss issues. The dedicated staff at the Medicare Rights Center, knowledgeable Capital Hill staffers, and beneficiaries I have encountered over the years have kept me grounded in reality. Many others have inspired me through their work and the help they have given me over time. I also want especially to thank my colleague and friend, Judy Feder, who makes me laugh, keeps me sane, and upon whom I rely for critical policy insights. Finally, Douglas Gomery, whose own work is an inspiration, pushes me to be better than I think I can be while steadfastly defending me to the rest of the world.

1

THE BENEFICIARY'S PERSPECTIVE

Medicare has contributed substantially to the well-being of America's oldest and most disabled citizens. The largest public health care program in the United States, Medicare provides the major source of acute care insurance for elderly and disabled populations. For some, Medicare represents a model of what national health insurance could be in the United States. With low administrative costs, the program is popular with both beneficiaries and the general population. At the same time, Medicare is one of the fastest growing programs in the federal budget, gobbling up new resources at the rate of 12 percent each year during its first 37 years. Critics assail the program as being out of sync with the needs of many senior citizens for failing to provide comprehensive services, while others often refer to it as "unsustainable" because of high costs. Physicians and hospital administrators endlessly criticize and debate Medicare, but rely upon it for a substantial share of their revenues.

This book examines the current status of Medicare and offers options for reform, with a particular focus on the program's beneficiaries: What is Medicare, how does it work, and where is it headed? What are the problems facing the program, and how can they be resolved? What options for the future hold the most promise? And most important, can current and future beneficiaries count on this program to be there for them? To understand the many different pressures on Medicare, it is useful to first examine the program from the perspective of the beneficiaries it serves (this chapter) and then look at it in the broader context of health care, the federal government, and the economy (chapter 2). Later chapters explore the history of Medicare, how the program works, and how it might change. Throughout, however, the intent is to emphasize the impacts on beneficiaries rather than on other players in the health care maze.

MEDICARE'S OFTEN OVERLOOKED SUCCESS

In examining Medicare, it is tempting to focus on the program's inadequacies, losing sight of Medicare's substantial accomplishments. But what works and works well must be kept in mind as changes to Medicare are contemplated. Reforms in Medicare need to protect its essential and most valuable elements.

Since the program first enrolled beneficiaries in 1966, almost all persons age 65 and over—and later, a substantial number of persons with disabilities—gained access to most doctors, hospitals, and other providers of health care services. Medicare almost immediately doubled the share of people age 65 and over with insurance. Before Medicare, only half of all older Americans had insurance (Andersen, Lion, and Anderson 1976). By 1970, 97 percent of older Americans were enrolled, and that proportion has remained about the same ever since (Moon 1996). Including the disabled, Medicare now reaches over 42 million people. It remains one of the most popular public programs and gets higher marks from its beneficiaries than do most private health insurance companies serving the younger population (Davis, Schoen, et al. 2002).

Two impacts followed immediately from Medicare's introduction: use of services by the population grew and financial burdens on older Americans and their families declined. Access to care increased, particularly for those who previously lacked the resources to obtain services. Although Medicare's benefit package has changed little since 1965, the program has stayed current in the service areas it covers. For example, many surgeries that once were performed on an inpatient basis are now performed on an outpatient basis, but since both inpatient and outpatient hospital care are covered, this transfer occurred without difficulty. Today, even the oldest Americans have access to mainstream medical care. New technology is available to beneficiaries, and, in some cases, new procedures are disseminated more quickly for the old than for the young (Moon 1999). Medicare's role was important for improving access and sped the desegregation of hospitals and other medical facilities by ensuring not only that minority seniors would receive care but that minorities of all ages could go to facilities previously closed to them. It is easy to forget that in 1965, for example, many black Americans could not go to the best hospitals, particularly in the South (Height 1996; Stevens 1996).

Financial burdens for seniors also fell nearly in half as a result of Medicare's introduction. Over time, the share of income that seniors spend on health care has crept back up, but their burdens would be much greater without Medicare. In 1965, the typical elderly person spent about 19 percent of her income on health care. That share fell to about 11 percent in 1968. In 2004, Medicare's contribution to the costs of health care for seniors totaled over $6,670, nearly 46 percent of the median income of persons age 65 and over (Boards of Trustees 2005). So, without Medicare, most of those now covered would pay more for their care, and many people would likely have to cut back on the amount of care they receive.

Finally, life expectancy since 1965 has improved at a faster pace for persons age 65 and over than for the population as a whole. In 1960, women faced a life expectancy at age 65 of 15.8 years; by 2001, that figure was 19.4 years. For men, life expectancy increased over the same period from 12.8 to 16.4 years (NCHS 2003). Some of this improvement is undoubtedly a byproduct of Medicare and Medicaid.

A Basic Primer on Medicare

Medicare offers two types of insurance options. The first is the traditional fee-for-service approach in which the government serves as the insurer. This is the "default" option—that is, beneficiaries are enrolled in this portion of the program unless they specifically opt to rely on a private plan for their benefits. The private plan option, Medicare Advantage, serves beneficiaries who wish to get their care through a private insurer, usually a managed care plan like a health maintenance organization (HMO). Persons age 65 and over who are eligible for any type of Social Security benefit, those receiving Social Security disability benefits for two years, and persons with end-stage renal disease (ESRD) are eligible for Medicare. While the program is briefly described here, it is outlined in more detail in appendix A.

Traditional Fee-for-Service

Under traditional Medicare, the federal government acts as an insurance company and bears the risk for the costs of the basic benefit package. This part of Medicare is divided into Parts A and B, reflecting the original split in financing for the program. In 2006, a new Part D benefit will be added to offer coverage for prescription drugs. Part A,

Hospital Insurance, is funded by payroll taxes and a portion of the taxation of Social Security benefits. It covers inpatient hospital care, skilled nursing benefits, hospice services, and some home health care. Part B, Supplementary Medical Insurance, is funded jointly by beneficiary-paid premiums and general revenues (mainly personal income taxes). Part B covers ambulatory services, including physician and related services; outpatient hospital care; and some home health care. Part A is available at no charge to those who qualify, and Part B is voluntary and requires a premium from enrollees—although the subsidy from general revenues is sufficiently generous to attract nearly all those eligible. Part D, Prescription Drug Insurance, will also be voluntary and will offer prescription drug coverage to those who enroll in a private plan established for this purpose. It will be financed in the same manner as Part B.

Part C, Medicare Advantage, is the private plan option portion. Individuals may choose to have private plans that participate in Medicare provide their benefits. Private plans are required to pay all benefits covered under A and B, and in 2006 to offer, as an option, a drug benefit. Beneficiaries who enroll usually must pay the Part B premium, and, in some cases, a premium for the extra services offered by private plans.

The premium for an individual who chooses to enroll in Part B is set at 25 percent of the average costs of Part B services for elderly beneficiaries.[1] Traditional fee-for-service Medicare also requires that individuals pay deductibles and coinsurance. Both Parts A and B have deductibles and most of the services are subject to some type of coinsurance (table 1.1). The Part A deductible ($912 in 2005) is particularly high. Part B's deductible is set much lower at $110 per year. The highest source of beneficiary costs come from coinsurance assessed against most Part B benefits. And there is no limit on the total that any one beneficiary might have to pay. As a consequence, beneficiaries were liable for about 26 percent of the overall costs of Medicare-covered services in 2004. In addition, a number of services, particularly vision and dental care, are not part of the basic benefit package. Most prescription drugs will not be added until 2006. As of 2005, the basic benefits offered do not comprise a comprehensive health insurance package. Medicare itself meets only 54 percent of beneficiaries' health care costs (Federal Interagency Forum on Aging-Related Statistics 2004).

When Medicare and its benefit package were created in 1965, medical care needs and insurance looked very different than they do today. For example, many workers had only hospital coverage, in part because health care spending as a share of income was much smaller, and expenses such as physician services were not inordinately expensive. Today, most good insurance plans for workers cover almost all aspects

Table 1.1. Cost-Sharing Requirements in Traditional Medicare, 2006

Requirement		2006 amounts
PART A		
Inpatient	Deductible	$952 per illness spell
	Co-payment for days 61–90	$238 per day
	Co-payment for lifetime reserve days 91–150	$476 per day
	Co-payment beyond day 150	100% of costs
Skilled Nursing Facility Care	Co-payment for days 21–100	Up to $119 per day
	Co-payment beyond 100 days	100% of costs
Home Health Care	Coinsurance for durable medical equipment	At least 20% of approved amount
Hospice	Co-payment for outpatient drugs	$5
	Coinsurance for inpatient respite care	5% of payment amount
Blood	First 3 pints	100% of costs
PART B		
	Premium	$88.50 per month
	Deductible	$124 per year
	Coinsurance	20% of charges

Source: Center for Medicare and Medicaid Services (2006).

of acute care, including generous drug coverage. Yet the basic package for Medicare remained largely unchanged until December 2003, when a new drug benefit option was enacted as part of the Medicare Prescription Drug, Improvement, and Modernization Act of 2003 (MMA). For example, one study found that 82 percent of employer-based plans had more generous health benefits than does Medicare (Hewitt Associates 2000). When Part D is added, Medicare's comprehensiveness will improve but only modestly. At that point, beneficiaries will be liable for about half the costs of their drug expenses on average and in 2006 will pay a premium of about $35 per month if they choose to enroll. As a consequence, Medicare's share of acute care spending will likely rise to about 58 percent.

Supplemental Plans

It is not surprising that a market for supplemental insurance developed soon after Medicare passed. Two types of private supplemental policies have evolved: employer-based retiree insurance and individual supplemental coverage (referred to as Medigap). Medicaid, a public benefit established at the same time as Medicare, subsidizes many low-income beneficiaries. These various plans cover services beyond the basic coverage Medicare provides, but they vary in quality, accessibility, and how much financial burden they relieve. Sometimes they simply fill in the coverage gaps from required deductibles and co-payments.

In 2001, approximately 33 percent of beneficiaries had employer-subsidized insurance and 28 percent had Medigap coverage. About 12 percent of beneficiaries receive help from the joint federal and state Medicaid program (Medicare Payment Advisory Commission [MedPAC] 2004b) (figure 1.1).

Employer-Based Plans. Employer-based plans normally offer comprehensive supplemental insurance. Employers usually pay for part of the premiums for this private coverage and, by filling in gaps left by Medicare, establish benefits comparable to what their working population receives. A large share of these plans, for example, cover prescription drugs. These plans reduce out-of-pocket expenses and increase access to services, often without limiting provider choice. Beneficiaries in these plans have among the lowest out-of-pocket costs of all Medicare beneficiaries (MedPAC 2002). But such plans are limited to workers and dependents whose former employers offer generous retiree benefits.[2] As a consequence, these benefits accrue mainly to higher-income

Figure 1.1. Sources of Supplemental Coverage among Noninstitutionalized Medicare Beneficiaries, 2001

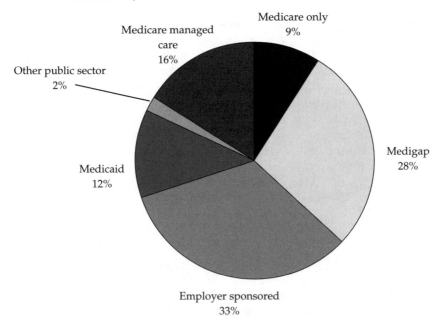

Source: Medicare Payment Advisory Commission (2004b).

retirees. Further, employers have reduced their liabilities by shifting more costs to retirees and reducing future promises of retiree health coverage (Henry J. Kaiser Family Foundation and Hewitt Associates 2004). Promised coverage for retirees is declining, although current Medicare beneficiaries are only beginning to feel the impacts of those changes.

Medigap. A traditional form of private supplemental coverage, commonly referred to as Medigap, leaves the financing burden on individuals since they usually pay full price for this coverage. Reforms in the early 1990s created 10 standardized plans that insurance companies may offer, covering a basic package of Medicare's required cost-sharing and in some cases including a limited prescription drug benefit.[3] The goal of this legislation was to make price comparisons easier for beneficiaries.

As a result of higher costs, even the limited drug coverage specified in three of the standard packages became more difficult to obtain after the mid-1990s, when drug costs began to rise. Many insurers have dropped such coverage or set prices so high that few can afford them. In 1998, only about 500,000 policies with prescription drugs were issued (MedPAC 2000), and the numbers have likely dropped since then. So Medigap mainly fills in the deductible and coinsurance charges for Medicare-covered services.

Further, since beneficiaries pay for the full costs of such insurance, including substantial administrative and marketing charges—and often, profits for the insurer—beneficiaries have mostly *greater*, not lower, financial burdens when they buy Medigap. Enrollees in these plans usually pay at least 120 percent of the actuarial value of the benefits (GAO 1998). Like all insurance, Medigap reduces potential catastrophic expenses for those who have high costs in a particular year. It smoothes out health care costs over time. But because Medigap policies tend to cover nearly the first dollar of expenditures, premiums are particularly high. Nonetheless, Medigap remains popular because Medicare offers no upper bound on potential liability for cost sharing.

Medigap premiums rose dramatically in the 1990s, though reliable national numbers are hard to find since prices vary considerably around the country. Between 1992 and 1996, premium rates in Arizona, Ohio, and Virginia rose 18, 41, and 19 percent, respectively, though the majority of those rate increases took place between 1995 and 1996 (Alexcih et al. 1997). National estimates for rate increases from 1999 to 2001 were 13 percent annually (Chollet 2003). Weiss Ratings (2003) reported that prices rose by 10.9 percent in 2001 and by just 2.4 percent in 2002. In general, these numbers resemble the patterns of Medicare spending but often exceed Medicare's actual growth rates.

Over time, Medigap plans have changed their pricing strategies, also contributing to access issues. Medigap providers can sell policies that are community-rated (i.e., the same for everyone) or that vary by age of beneficiary (Alexcih et al. 1997). Companies have moved away from community-rated plans, where the premium is the same for all those enrolled each year in a particular plan. Most providers have moved to an "attained-age" structure in which policies increase in cost rapidly as people age. This puts greater burdens on Medicare beneficiaries just as their incomes decline. For the unwary buyer at age 65, these plans appear less costly than community-rated options. But after the six-month period of open enrollment at age 65, underwriting makes it difficult for beneficiaries to change Medigap plans. So beneficiaries who choose policies that are inexpensive at first may get locked into policies that become increasingly expensive as they age. An option to offer lower-cost Medigap plans was added in 1997 when legislation established a high deductible option for those wishing mainly to obtain supplemental catastrophic protection. That has not proven to be popular either with insurers or enrollees, however (Fox et al. 2003). For insurers, the lower premiums associated with high deductible plans likely lower their potential profits while they still must track total spending. And Medicare beneficiaries have traditionally preferred comprehensive gap-filling policies.

Medicaid. Medicaid, which offers generous fill-in benefits for Medicare, is limited to persons with low incomes. Medicaid is a joint federal and state program in which states have some latitude in establishing eligibility and coverage. At the discretion of the state, basic Medicaid coverage is generally limited to people with incomes well below the federal poverty level—often at or below 74 percent of the poverty level (Holahan and Pohl 2003). For those who get these benefits, coverage is usually comprehensive. In addition to paying Medicare's Part B premium and relieving beneficiaries of the responsibility for co-payments and deductibles, traditional Medicaid offers prescription drug coverage, long-term care, and other services, although the details vary by state. Low rates of payments to care providers, however, may affect access to services. Most states also offer a medically needy program, allowing individuals with higher incomes to participate if they have substantial health expenditures. Many elderly and disabled who reside in institutions achieve Medicaid eligibility in this way. In both cases, individuals must also have very few assets to qualify.[4]

The programs added since 1988 provide additional relief for low-income Medicare beneficiaries and together are referred to as the Medicare Savings programs. The Qualified Medicare Beneficiary Program (QMB), covers Part B premiums, deductibles, and coinsurance for people whose incomes fall below 100 percent of the poverty level (about $8,950 in 2004 for a single person). The Specified Low-Income Medicare Beneficiary (SLMB) program provides Part B premium subsidies for those with incomes between 100 and 120 percent of the poverty level. Finally, the 1997 Balanced Budget Act created the Qualified Individuals (QI) program to cover the full premium costs for people with incomes between 120 and 135 percent of the poverty level (QI1) and a small portion of premium costs for those up to 175 percent of the poverty level (QI2) (Moon, Gage, and Evans 1997). The QI2 benefits, which were never broadly used, expired in 2002.

In practice, standard Medicaid and the Medicare Savings programs cover only some people who qualify for them. Traditional Medicaid, for example, only covers about half of all persons with incomes below the poverty level. In 1996, only 55 percent of those eligible participated in QMB, and just 16 percent of those eligible participate in SLMB (Barents Group 1999). The relationship to welfare and the complexity of the application process are often cited as reasons for low participation (Medicare Rights Center 2002). The rationale for appending the Medicare Savings programs to Medicaid rather than Medicare was to prevent any appearance of treating Medicare as a means-tested program. More recently, low participation rates have caused some policymakers to consider making these protections a formal part of Medicare. The low-income protections for the new drug benefit extend eligibility to 150 percent of the poverty level but have an asset requirement. Nonetheless, this new low-income protection is formally part of Medicare.

When thinking about policy from a beneficiary's perspective, it is important to keep these public supplemental benefits in mind. They can help to fill in gaps, but the low participation rates (likely because of the welfare nature of Medicaid) and the limited benefits they provide above 100 percent of the poverty level mean that low-income protection for Medicare beneficiaries still leaves much to be desired.

Medicare Advantage

The second part of Medicare is now referred to as Medicare Advantage (MA). Established in the 2003 legislation, MA replaced the previous managed care option (called Medicare + Choice between 1997 and 2003) with a set of reforms that changed how private plans are paid and established. Both the 1997 and 2003 reforms were attempts to foster private sector alternatives to the traditional, public fee-for-service Medicare option. The federal government contracts with private insurers—so far, mostly health maintenance organizations (HMOs)—to cover all Medicare benefits (i.e., both Parts A and B) for a fixed monthly payment. Beneficiaries then get their Medicare benefits through these private insurance plans, which bear the risk for the costs of care.

Most of these plans offer some additional benefits, such as lower cost-sharing requirements. And in the 1990s, prescription drugs and other noncovered services were offered with no or only modest premiums beyond the Part B premium. The years 1999 and 2000 were the "golden age" of private plans; plan and enrollee participation has declined since that time, but increased in 2004 and 2005 in response to changes from legislation in late 2003. Nonetheless, enrollment remains below its earlier peak levels. While the 1997 legislation sought to encourage more types of plans to enroll, it also slowed the growth in payments to plans. This slowdown was legislated because evidence indicated that Medicare plans were overpaid (GAO 2000); nonetheless, the response by plans was dramatic, with many plan withdrawals and a decline in the share of beneficiaries enrolled from 16 percent of the beneficiary population in 1999 to 11 percent in 2003 (figure 1.2) (Boards of Trustees 2005). Since then it has risen to about 13 percent of the population.

Most plans that did not withdraw from participating in Medicare limited additional benefits or raised the premiums they charged. The plans became less attractive to beneficiaries seeking lower out-of-pocket costs (Gold and Achman 2003). By 2003, not only were the numbers of plans and beneficiaries at low levels, enrollment was concentrated in only a few states. For example, enrollment in Medicare + Choice exceeded 30 percent of beneficiaries in California, Oregon, and Rhode Island, but 16 states had no enrollees (CMS 2004b).

The 2003 prescription drug legislation added generous new payments to private plans, starting in 2004, to once again encourage them to

Figure 1.2. Yearly Enrollment in Medicare Advantage Plan

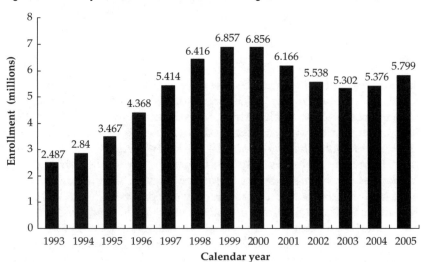

Source: Boards of Trustees (2005).

participate in Medicare. Estimates of these increased payments indicate that private plans receive about 8 percent more than it would cost to serve beneficiaries in traditional fee-for-service Medicare (Biles, Nicholas, and Cooper 2004). This differential is over and above the advantages that private plans have had because they serve a healthier-than-average population.[5] It is too early to tell how much difference these higher payments are likely to make over time, but after one year, participation in such plans has increased by over 400,000 (Gold and Harris 2005). This complicated relationship between Medicare and private plans will be described in more detail in chapter 5.

Supplemental Coverage Issues

When thinking about policy changes in Medicare, it is important to consider the complexities that supplemental policies create. Beneficiaries grouped by supplemental coverage are likely to view coverage expansions differently. For example, the approximately one-third of beneficiaries with employer-subsidized coverage have the most comprehensive benefits and may see little need for expanding Medicare, particularly if they have to pay for the expansion. And these beneficiaries often fear, as they did with the new drug legislation, that expansions in Medicare coverage will cause employers to cut benefits. About one-fourth of beneficiaries have Medicaid or Medicare Advantage coverage, both of which offer additional benefits, although both may be subject to cuts in the future. From government's point of view, expanded benefits to beneficiaries in Medicaid or Medicare are likely to be at least partially offset by lower government costs elsewhere. That is, improving basic Medicare benefits would help states that spend a substantial share of their Medicaid dollars on filling in the gaps in coverage from basic Medicare (and there would be offsetting reductions in federal spending on Medicaid contributions as well). Medicare Advantage plans, which have successfully obtained higher payments from the federal government, will likely reinstate some of the extra benefits that they reduced in the early 2000s and perhaps again attract more beneficiaries. In 2004, for example, plans used about half their increased payments to raise benefits. But later in this decade, cost cutting may again reduce payment generosity, leading to the same incentives to retrench as seen at the turn of the century.

But for the remaining third of beneficiaries who rely on Medigap or who have no supplemental coverage, expansions are extremely important and would likely reduce out-of-pocket costs considerably. Beneficiaries who cannot afford to purchase supplemental coverage and who are not eligible for Medicaid are the most vulnerable to high out-of-pocket costs. Since they are likely to be older and poorer, high Medicare out-of-pocket costs likely prevent them from getting needed care. And the increasingly high costs of Medigap also put those beneficiaries at risk. Some of the very old are dropping their plans, for example, as premiums continue to rise.

ECONOMIC STATUS OF MEDICARE BENEFICIARIES

A key factor in considering changes in Medicare is the impact, mostly financial, on beneficiaries. Are beneficiaries able to absorb substantially higher cost sharing or premiums, for example? Should older Americans' improved well-being affect their special treatment in a government program? Will they be substantially better off in the near future? These questions need to be front and center before considering how the program should change. Furthermore, the situations of persons 65 and older differ from the under-65 disabled population and merit separate consideration. And if costs rise for vulnerable groups among Medicare beneficiaries, these financial issues can translate into problems accessing care.

The Economic Status of Older Beneficiaries

By every measure of economic well-being, the situation for older Americans has improved substantially over the past four decades. But the overall level remains modest and the diversity in economic status still leaves many behind in terms of financial health.[6]

Income. Income for people 65 and older has risen steadily from a median per capita income of $3,408 in 1975 to $14,664 in 2003 (U.S. Bureau of the Census 1991, 2004).[7] After controlling for inflation, this represents a gain of 26 percent in the purchasing power of this age group over approximately 30 years. Although seniors have made some gains relative to the young, particularly during the 1970s, per capita median income is still lower for older Americans than for younger adults. In 2003, median income per capita for persons age 18 to 64 was $26,117, compared with $14,664 for seniors.

However, to comprehend fully the ability of elderly individuals to meet their needs, it is crucial to look beyond income and to understand the diversity of resources available to this group. Although the elderly have shown impressive gains overall, not every older individual has shared in the rosier economic status. For example, some of the increase in well-being associated with comparisons of incomes across time reflects the changing composition of the elderly. Each year, individuals turning age 65 join the elderly category, and the incomes of new 65-year-olds tend, on average, to be higher each year. But individuals within the elderly population display slower rates of income growth than does the group as a whole because the overall group's composition is changing as younger, higher-income groups replace lower-income decedents. To illustrate, figure 1.3 shows median incomes for persons age 65 through 69 in 1983 and then follows that cohort through time, documenting the decline in per capita income for people as they age. If instead the focus is on 65- to 69-year-olds in each identified time period, the comparisons made across years show greater growth that reflects the improvement in economic status of each new cohort in that age range. This sometimes results in the conclusion that seniors are better off than ever—something often not the case for a specific cohort.

What about elderly persons with substantial resources? This is the group that many policymakers would target for cuts in Medicare benefits. As figure 1.4 indicates, less than 10 percent of seniors had per capita incomes above $50,000 in 2003. More than two-thirds of seniors are concentrated in the income categories below $25,000. So, if the focus is on "Warren Buffet" or "Bill Gates's father" as some pundits argue, the number of Medicare beneficiaries subject to scrutiny would be very small indeed. Seniors with per capita incomes above $100,000 total only about 2 percent of all people age 65 and over. And since the

Figure 1.3. Real Per Capita Income of Selected Age Groups ($)

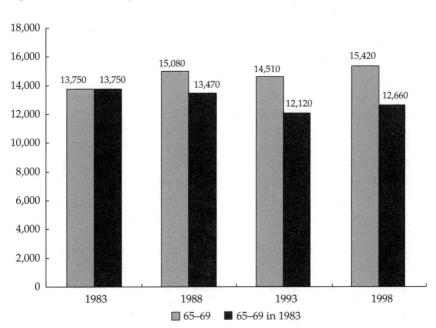

Sources: Current Population Survey, March Supplement (1984, 1989, 1994, 1999).

Figure 1.4. Distribution of Per Capita Income of Elderly, 2003

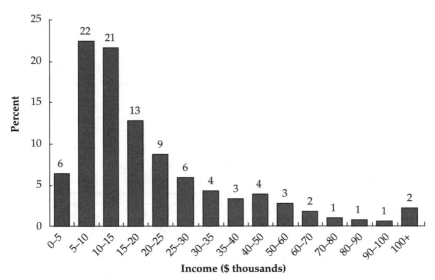

Source: Current Population Survey (2004).

debate in the 2004 presidential election over whether to eliminate tax cuts for the wealthy often referred to $200,000 as the income cutoff for the upper middle class, it is difficult to make the claim that older Americans today are "well off."

Finally, when evaluating the incomes of the elderly, it is important to remember that income inequality has been widening for all age groups since the late 1970s. Incomes for the low-income elderly have been growing, but at lower rates than incomes for the high-income elderly (U.S. Congress, Committee of Ways and Means 1994; Clark et al. 2004). Sources of income grow at different rates. For example, people with lower overall incomes depend more heavily on Social Security and other public programs that tend to just keep up with inflation. Those with income from wages and from stocks, bonds, and other investments generally have enjoyed more rapid income growth over time.

In sum, the dichotomy between the wealthiest and the poorest elderly Medicare beneficiaries has grown over time, creating new challenges for public policy. Should the highest income elderly, for example, contribute substantially more to the costs of their care? The answer hinges on society's judgment on a variety of issues, but key among them are how well-off we perceive older persons to be relative to younger

Americans and whether the "rich" constitute a large enough group to merit inordinate attention.

Poverty. Elderly poverty has declined over time, though not by as much as some would argue. The share of the elderly in poverty dropped from 25 percent in 1968 to 10.2 percent in 2003 (U.S. Bureau of the Census 1995, 2004). These rates declined rapidly through 1975, then declined slowly through 1995 and have shown little change since then. Measures of poverty are derived by comparing family incomes against defined poverty cutoff or threshold levels, which vary by family size. These are the thresholds above which people can meet at least basic subsistence needs. Such a measure is often useful when making comparisons across age groups because it controls for the fact that family size is generally smaller for older Americans than for families headed by persons age 35 to 64, for example. In 2003, the U.S. Census defined an individual 65 and over living alone as poor if his or her income fell below $8,825 in 2003. The cutoff level for a couple was $11,122.

Determining exactly what the poverty cutoff level should be remains controversial. For example, the U.S. Department of Health and Human Services uses a different set of poverty guidelines for determining eligibility for public programs that increases the proportion of elderly persons reported as poor. Further, an extensive analysis of poverty measures by the National Research Council (1995) concluded that health care costs should be more explicitly included in a measure of poverty for older Americans, which would also create a higher poverty standard. The implications of these measurement issues are discussed in appendix B.

All of these alternative numbers point to substantial improvement in poverty rates since Medicare passed in 1965. For many seniors, however, the improvements have not resulted in *substantial* increases in living standards. A large number of older persons have incomes just above the official Census poverty line, leaving them extremely vulnerable if not technically poor. In 2003, 3.6 million individuals 65 or older were listed as poor using the standard Census measure. Another 2.3 million had incomes of no more than 25 percent above the poverty threshold. This 125 percent figure is often used instead of 100 percent, given criticism about the inadequacy of the measure (figure 1.5). Using that figure, improvements over time have been more modest. When we count the total number with incomes below 150 percent of the poverty threshold, 24.6 percent of the elderly—about 8.5 million persons—had very limited incomes in 2001 (U.S. Bureau of the Census 2004). Affordability of Medicare benefits continues to be a substantial issue for elderly beneficiaries.

Assets and Net Worth. It is true that the elderly hold more assets, on average, than other families with low and moderate incomes. But

Figure 1.5. Persons Age 65 and Over with Incomes Below 100 and 125 Percent of Census Poverty Threshold

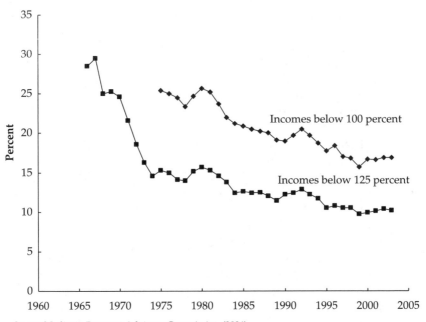

Source: Medicare Payment Advisory Commission (2004).

even if assets were incorporated into poverty measures, only a small share of the poor would have their financial status boosted to any major degree (Moon, Friedland, and Shirey 2002). The dollar values are higher when housing is included, but even in that case, median asset holdings for elderly households in 2000 totaled $108,885 and just $23,369 when home equity is excluded (U.S. Bureau of the Census 2003).

Forty percent of all Medicare beneficiaries had financial assets of less than $12,000, and more than 80 percent of those with incomes below 175 percent of the poverty level had less than $12,000 in assets (Moon et al. 2002). It is simply not true that older persons who are "income poor" are "asset rich" and hence living very well.

However, assets do help supplement income for many retirees with above average incomes and add to their economic well-being. In fact, older persons are increasingly retiring with financial assets they have accumulated to meet their retirement needs. These funds are often available in lieu of a pension. IRAs and 401Ks, for example, may initially appear as large amounts of assets, but need to be spread across retirement years. Indeed, assets should be considered not resources for any one year, but lifetime support that retirees can receive either through formally purchasing an annuity or gradually spending principal. For example, using a standard annuity formula, a woman age 70 with assets of $12,000 could increase her income by $914 per year if she allocated it evenly over the rest of her life. This asset level is twice as high as the eligibility cutoff for extra protection for the new drug benefit, even though it increases available resources by only a modest amount.

Sources of Income for the Elderly. Older Americans rely on a broad range of resources (figure 1.6). For those outside the labor force, Social Security remains the major component of income for most seniors. For one-third of seniors, Social Security constitutes over 90 percent of their incomes (Grad 2003), and for nearly two-thirds, it makes up over half their incomes. Traditionally, Social Security represents a strong and reliable base for incomes in retirement. Ad hoc increases in the 1960s and early 1970s help explain much of the decline in poverty. And since cost-of-living adjustments were added after 1972, benefits keep pace with inflation, and older persons are assured of not living beyond their resources. However, as debates on Social Security's future continue to

Figure 1.6. Sources of Income for Elderly

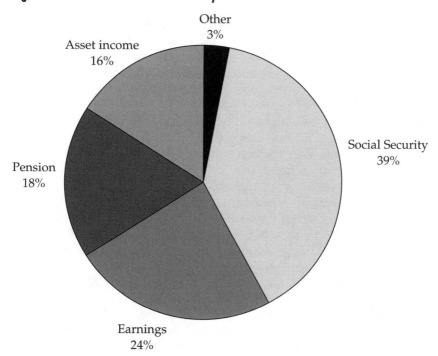

Source: Grad (2003).

take place, the uncertainty surrounding this source of income raises key issues for Medicare and its affordability for future retirees. Projections of seniors' incomes over time have assumed that Social Security will be there in the future. But if benefits are cut or if benefits depend on stock market and other investment returns, some future Medicare beneficiaries may have difficulty meeting their increasing health care costs. At the least, the inequality of incomes is likely to rise.

Older Americans fortunate enough to have income from pensions are generally concentrated in the upper income ranges. For example, while pensions account for 18 percent of incomes on average for the aged, they account for only 3 percent of the incomes for those in the bottom fifth of the income distribution (figure 1.7) (Grad 2003). For those in the top 20 percent of income, pensions accounted for 20 percent. This source of income has remained relatively constant over time but is expected to decline as fewer individuals receive traditional pensions in the future. Instead, many Americans will be covered by defined contribution plans that do not guarantee a certain benefit each month. That is, employees and their employers make contributions that are invested in the stock market and elsewhere. The amount available at retirement is dependent upon how well the individual has done with these investments. Again, this may increase some of the inequality in well-being over time.

Many Medicare beneficiaries have high incomes because they continue to rely on wages. Actually, wage earners among the elderly tend to represent two categories: individuals with enjoyable high-end jobs and those whose retirement resources are so low that they feel they must remain in the labor force indefinitely. Certainly these are two very different groups of individuals, which likely need to be thought of quite differently. Many high-end workers have employer-based health insurance and rely on that rather than on Medicare for most of their health needs. Low-wage workers, however, often have no private insurance and, like other retirees, may be relying on Medigap or Medicare Advantage to supplement Medicare.

For people with the lowest incomes, the Supplemental Security Income program offers a means-tested benefit to bring individuals up closer to the poverty lines. But unless the state in which the individual resides offers supplemental benefits, the basic benefit is not enough to raise a person up to or above the poverty level. About 5 percent of elderly Medicare beneficiaries rely on SSI to supplement their incomes. As the poorest of Medicare beneficiaries, those with SSI are automatically enrolled in the Medicaid program, which does a good job of supplementing their health care needs, though the generosity of coverage and access to care can depend on their state of residence. These and other "dual eligibles" with access to both Medicare and Medicaid

Figure 1.7. Sources of Income for Elderly at Bottom and Top of Income Distribution

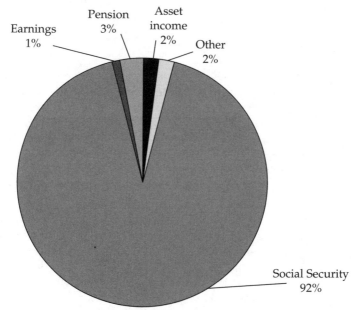

**Households in bottom
20% of income**

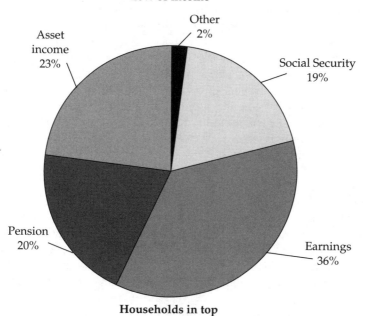

**Households in top
20% of income**

Source: Grad (2003).

are discussed in more detail later in this chapter when examining the burdens that out-of-pocket costs impose on Medicare beneficiaries.

The Economic Status of Disabled Persons

Medicare is usually seen as a program for the over-65 population, and much of the focus on changes in the program considers that population's ability to pay for its own health care. But Medicare also covers younger disabled Americans. In fact, the numbers of such beneficiaries increased dramatically in the 1990s. The younger disabled totaled 6.4 million in 2004 and constituted over 15 percent of all Medicare beneficiaries, compared with less than 10 percent in 1990 (CMS 2004a). The economic status of disabled Medicare beneficiaries is much less well studied than that of the elderly, however.

Individuals must receive Social Security Disability Insurance (DI) benefits for a total of two years before Medicare coverage begins, and since there is a five-month waiting period for DI, new beneficiaries must have been disabled for 29 months. Under the Social Security definition of disability, an individual must be unable to engage in substantial gainful activity because of a medically determinable physical or mental impairment expected to last at least 12 months or until death. In addition to disabled workers, disabled widow(er)s and disabled adult children of workers are eligible to participate. (However, family members of DI beneficiaries are not eligible for Medicare.)

By definition, such individuals must be unable to work, so unless other family members are in the labor force, the family is likely to face severe economic constraints. The onset of disability may occur in conjunction with high levels of spending on medical care and high rates of absenteeism from the workplace. Both of these factors may drain the resources of a disabled worker and family. Disabled persons must then wait for two years after qualifying for Social Security benefits to become eligible for benefits. If they had employee-sponsored coverage, they are allowed to continue in that plan but must pay its full premium costs.

One early study found that disabled Social Security recipients were more likely to be poor compared with either the general population or persons receiving Social Security as retired workers (Grad 1989).[7] The rate of poverty was 19 percent for these disabled persons, and an additional 11 percent were near poor. By comparison, only 17 percent of retired workers were poor or near poor during that same period. By 1996, these factors had changed very little. Medicare disabled beneficiaries have, on average, significantly lower personal incomes than elderly beneficiaries. That is, in 1996, 27 percent of all families with a disabled Medicare beneficiary had incomes of less than $10,000 compared to 16.7 percent of families with an elderly beneficiary. And nearly two-thirds of families with a disabled beneficiary had incomes of less than $25,000. The overall poverty rate for the disabled was 29.7 percent in 1996, compared with 11.2 percent for elderly beneficiaries (Henry J. Kaiser Family Foundation 2000).

Poverty rates of disabled beneficiaries vary substantially depending upon their living arrangements. Those most likely to be in poverty are disabled beneficiaries who live alone or with nonrelatives—and who have no other family members who work.[8] Over 48 percent of such beneficiaries live below the poverty line. This group represents 42 percent of all disabled beneficiaries. At a rate of 13.5 percent, disabled beneficiaries who are family heads or spouses of family heads constitute the group with the lowest level of poverty. However, they constitute just 17.4 percent of all disabled beneficiaries. The remaining 40.3 percent of disabled beneficiaries live with other relatives; 33.4 percent of them have incomes below the poverty cutoff (Kaiser 2000).

In 2002, median per capita incomes for disabled beneficiaries were just $9,420, compared with elderly Medicare beneficiaries whose per capita incomes were $14,476. Disabled workers are even less likely to have assets on which to draw than are their older counterparts, since the former have not had as many years or opportunities to accumulate wealth.

Despite potentially greater health needs, disabled beneficiaries are less likely than the elderly to have supplemental insurance. More than twice as many disabled beneficiaries as the elderly have no insurance beyond Medicare. Medigap insurance is often not available to disabled persons. For example, there is no federal guaranteed access to Medigap plans for the disabled, although elderly beneficiaries have such a guarantee during their first six months of Medicare eligibility. And proposals to make such insurance available to the disabled and add an open enrollment period for Medigap plans have not been enacted into law.

When the disabled do have additional coverage, it is more likely to come from the Medicaid program or from employer coverage through spouses or parents. Both these sources of protection are more important for the disabled than for persons age 65 and over. Indeed, 40.3 percent of disabled beneficiaries are dually eligible, compared with 13.4 percent of the elderly (CMS 2004a).

Burdens of Health Spending on Medicare Beneficiaries

As noted, the Medicare program covers only a portion of individuals' expenditures on health care, leaving a substantial amount to be paid out of pocket and resulting in a lower standard of living. The percentage of income spent on health care by Medicare beneficiaries reached an all-time high in 2005 and is expected to increase further. This spending represents a critical burden for Medicare beneficiaries. For example, about 23 percent of the incomes of elderly persons living in the community paid for their health care in 2004. For certain groups, the share is even higher (table 1.2). These figures have risen steadily over the years from 15 percent in 1987 to over 22 percent in 2004 (figure 1.8). Earlier estimates indicated that the share spent on acute health care services by older Americans would continue to rise from 22 percent in 2000 to

Table 1.2. Spending and Shares of Income Spent on Healthcare by Medicare Subgroups, 2004

Subgroups	Share of the population (%)	Out-of-pocket spending ($)	Out-of-pocket spending as a share of income (%)
Medicare Status			
Disabled	14.6	2,441	21.6
Elderly	85.4	3,274	22.8
65–69	23.5	2,731	17.0
70–79	40.7	3,483	23.8
80+	21.2	3,476	27.3
Gender			
Male	44.4	3,061	20.5
Female	55.6	3,226	24.4
Health Status			
Physical impairments	16.1	3,699	27.5
Cognitive impairments	13.3	2,725	21.8
Both impairments	9.5	3,447	30.8
None	61.1	3,056	20.2
Income as a Share of Poverty			
Less than or equal to 100%	17.5	2,357	41.3
101%–149%	17.1	2,987	29.5
150%–199%	12.1	3,218	25.0
200%–299%	19.6	3,249	18.7
300%+	33.6	3,572	10.9
Insurance Status			
Medicaid	11.3	2,305	29.9
Employer	40.2	3,025	16.8
Medigap	28.3	4,251	27.7
None	14.5	2,054	20.3
Total	100.0	3,152	24.7

Source: American Institutes for Research analysis of the 2000 Medicare Current Beneficiary Survey projected to 2004.

Note: Excludes institutionalized, ESRD, and HMO beneficiaries.

Figure 1.8. Out-of-Pocket Spending as a Share of Income among Elderly Beneficiaries

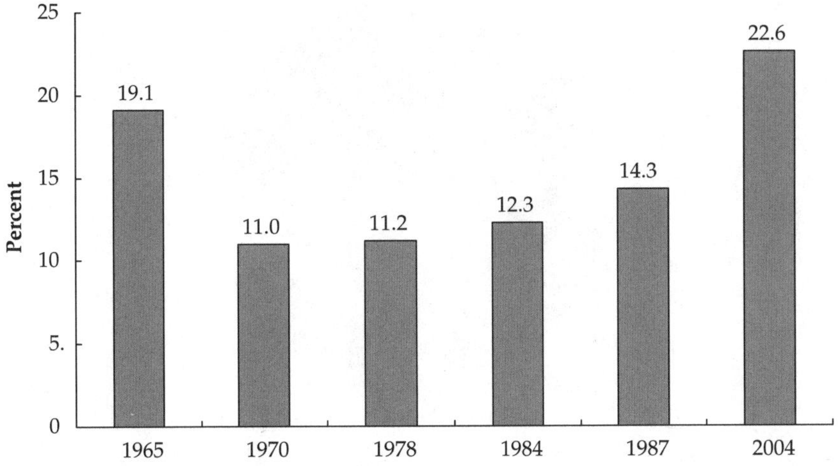

Source: Author's calculations.

about 30 percent of incomes by 2030 (Maxwell, Moon, and Segal 2001). That figure may prove to be too low given the higher 2004 share, caused in part by the rapid increase in the costs of prescription drugs. Incomes have risen for this age group, but out-of-pocket health costs have simply risen faster.

While most Medicare beneficiaries now have some type of supplemental coverage to help pay for health costs, that does not necessarily reduce the burden of paying for that care. In fact, when premiums are included in the calculation of out-of-pocket costs for Medicare beneficiaries (excluding those in institutions, enrolled in Medicare Advantage, and who have ESRD), premiums comprise a substantial share of what people spend each year on their health (figure 1.9).

In addition to the costs of acute health care spending, an important proportion of the Medicare population requires long-term care services.[9] The costs of long-term care hold the potential for devastating reductions in economic status for this population. For example, on average, elderly Medicare enrollees in the community spent $8,466 on health care compared with $46,810 for those in institutions (Federal Interagency Forum on Aging-Related Statistics 2004). The burdens these costs impose are hard to evaluate, but an individual pays, on average, more than $70,000 for a year's stay in a nursing home (Metlife Mature Market Institute 2004), and that amount can be much higher in certain parts of the country. Medicare pays for only a small share of long-term care, and Medicaid only covers these costs for people

Figure 1.9. Distribution of Out-of-Pocket Spending among Elderly Beneficiaries, 2004

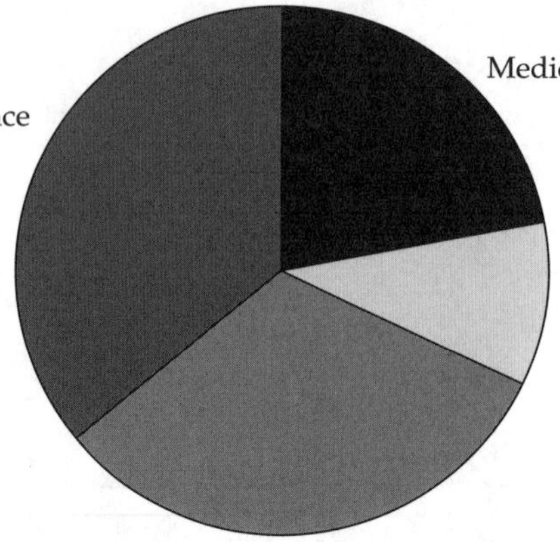

Medicare Part B premium
22%

Supplemental Insurance
premium
36%

Cost-sharing for
Medicare services
10%

Non-Medicare services
32%

Source: MedPAC (2004a).

with very low incomes or once individuals have spent down nearly all of their income and assets. Even with Medicaid protection to lessen the impact of this "spend down" on married couples, the spouse remaining in the community often faces a reduced standard of living. It is under these conditions that even middle-class elderly families find it financially impossible to meet their health care needs.

The likelihood of incurring costs from both acute and long-term health care rises steadily with age—in inverse proportion to ability to pay: an elderly woman living alone is most at risk of needing long-term care (Doty, Liu, and Wiener 1985). And the outlook for the future is not reassuring. Wiener, Illston, and Hanley (1994) suggest that only a minority of older families will ever be able to afford long-term care expenditures. Although this book does not deal directly with long-term care, it is important to remember that anything that reduces Medicare spending for the very old or those in poor health will likely exacerbate the financing issues facing those in need of long-term care.

The economic status of Medicare beneficiaries has improved considerably over time, but a key issue is whether the improvements will continue. If so, Medicare beneficiaries may be better able to handle health-spending demands, for example. But given past experience and future projections, burdens of health care will likely expand faster, for the foreseeable future, than Medicare beneficiaries' ability to pay. For example, over the same period that median incomes rose 26 percent, real out-of-pocket spending on health care more than doubled. The

Medicare actuaries have estimated that a 65-year-old beneficiary receiving a Social Security benefit equal to the average benefit for all OASDI beneficiaries will have 7.6 percent of that benefit taken out for the Part B premium (Sol Mussey, personal communication with Congressman Pete Stark, February 7, 2004). And if all Medicare liabilities were considered, they would account for 18.6 percent of the Social Security benefit in 2004. In 2010 (when drug costs are also included), this amount would rise to 39.2 percent of the Social Security benefit, and by 2030, 55.3 percent (figure 1.10). Since incomes of the elderly tend to rise at about the same rate as Social Security's annual increases, these shares of Social Security benefits offer a good indication of the likely impact of Medicare spending growing faster than incomes of the elderly.

BASIC ISSUES FACING FUTURE REFORMS

Sometimes lost in the enthusiasm to reform Medicare is a careful assessment of whether the original principles and goals for the program can and should be retained. Each raises questions that need to be revisited,

Figure 1.10. Medicare Liability as a Share of Social Security Benefit (Illustrative of 65- and 85-Year-Olds)

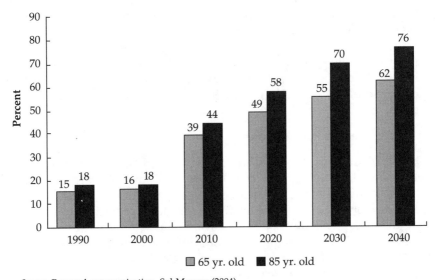

Source: Personal communication, Sol Mussey (2004).
Note: In 2010 and beyond, there is a large increase in liability because drugs become a Medicare benefit. If all out-of-pocket costs were shown, the share would be higher in earlier years.

with consideration for how well potential changes meet these basic protections for beneficiaries.

Mainstream Care

During the debate over Medicare's passage, a clear goal was to ensure that beneficiaries had access to mainstream care. With care providers expressing criticism and concern, there was reason to worry that Medicare would be considered a second-class program. Efforts to address this concern occurred on two levels: making the program operate like good private insurance policies and structuring Medicare so as to encourage health care providers to participate. The original legislation contained assurances about levels of payment and noninterference in the practice of medicine (Myers 1970).

This goal of providing access to mainstream care is often raised in two areas of reform discussions. First, is the benefit package adequate? Over the past 40 years, much has changed in what is covered in private-sector plans, making Medicare's coverage inadequate in comparison. The new prescription drug coverage will help but still will not bring Medicare beneficiaries' coverage to a level equal to workers' coverage.

Second, given the many changes in the nature of insurance in the private sector, would similar changes to Medicare be appropriate? The original goal of ensuring mainstream care was to provide access to high-quality care. Given the dissatisfaction with and decline of strict managed care in the private sector, "modernization" efforts to expand managed care through use of private programs may not improve Medicare. This has particularly become an issue as the private sector has moved away from managed care. Some policymakers advocate going even further by creating a voucher system where individuals would have to choose among private plans with limited subsidies from the government. Under such a plan, will everyone have mainstream care?

A Commitment to Pooling Risks

One of Medicare's accomplishments is that the very old and the very sick have access to the same basic benefits as younger, healthier beneficiaries. While there is certainly room for improvement, Medicare remains insurance that is never rescinded because of the individual's poor health. In fact, by expanding coverage to persons with disabilities in 1972, Medicare redoubled its commitment to insuring those who are most in need. Further, the premium for Part B, which is the contribution that most enrollees make while on Medicare, is the same for all beneficiaries regardless of age or health status (although an income-related premium is scheduled to begin in 2007).

In the private sector, even when there is a commitment to sharing risks, risk pooling at the same level as traditional Medicare is difficult to achieve. When individuals can move from plan to plan, plans face a strong incentive to seek those who are just a little healthier on average. In that way, plans can offer better services to their healthier clients for a given price. This is good for some enrollees, but the break-up in the risk pool can be extremely detrimental to persons with the greatest needs.

Consequently, the goal of risk pooling is likely to conflict with options to rely on private insurance plans that tailor their benefits to attract particular groups. By the nature of such options, the risk pool is split, and efforts to adjust for risk differences have fallen short. Do the advantages of private options outweigh the benefits of risk pooling?

Additional Help to Individuals in Need

By making Medicare a benefit available to all who qualify and setting contributions on the basis of ability to pay, Medicare also meets the principle of "social" insurance. When Medicare began, persons without insurance—the group most likely to gain from Medicare—tended to have lower incomes and be older. One of the reasons for a public commitment to health care for the elderly and disabled was to achieve some equality in services regardless of ability to pay.

This goal is now central to the current debate over expansion of benefits: should improvements be universal or limited to those with the fewest resources? Medicare was introduced as a universal program, even though some individuals would benefit more than others, as a way to achieve and retain broad support. Do the benefits of this approach justify the higher costs of a universal benefit compared with a more targeted one? On the other hand, a voucher approach that provides equal contributions to beneficiaries toward the cost of premiums may preclude persons with low incomes from accessing more expensive plan options; this could lead to a two-tiered Medicare program.

When the focus is on beneficiaries, it quickly becomes clear that their relatively modest economic resources, the high costs of health care, and diversity within the Medicare population indicate the need to improve Medicare. However, taxpayers' interests may not always lead in the same direction as beneficiaries' interests, as will become clear in chapter 2.

2

MEDICARE IN THE "BIG PICTURE"

Legislation to limit the size of Medicare reflects a desire to hold the line on government spending. In 2004, federal government spending on Medicare totaled $297 billion (Boards of Trustees 2005). It is the second largest federal domestic program, and in the last four decades, has often been the fastest growing part of the federal budget. Not surprisingly, in the 1980s through 1997, the federal government made Medicare a major focus of budget reduction efforts nearly every year. Substantial changes to Medicare under the Balanced Budget Act of 1997 (BBA) helped to achieve a balanced federal budget in 1998 for the first time in nearly 30 years.

Medicare, like the rest of health care spending, has grown at a rapid clip when measured as a share of gross domestic product (GDP). The addition of a drug benefit in 2006 means program spending will increase compared with GDP. And as the first members of the Baby Boom generation near age 65, Medicare promises to grow even faster beginning in 2011. But as figure 2.1 shows, the growth closely tracks the increase in the share of Americans receiving Medicare. Medicare has already doubled the number of persons it covers, and the numbers will double again by 2030. This doubling will substantially expand Medicare beneficiaries as a share of the total population.

Debate over Medicare will continue for the foreseeable future as financial pressures grow. This will happen no matter how important or essential the program is for helping seniors and disabled persons

Figure 2.1. Growth in Medicare Spending as a Share of GDP and in Beneficiaries as a Share of Total Population

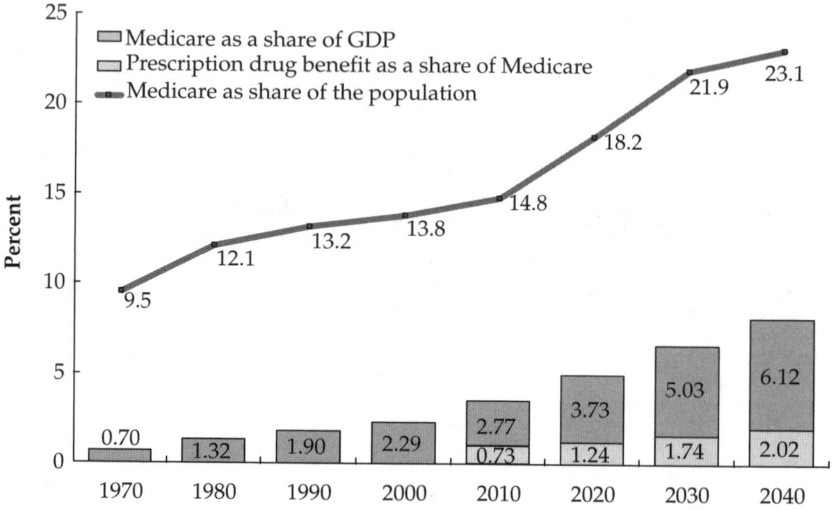

Sources: OASDI (2005), Medicare Trustees Report (2005).

obtain health care because these services receive public funds. However, it is important to put these issues in context. Is Medicare too large? How does it compare with our views as a society on health care spending and who should pay? The task of this chapter is to examine Medicare, its place in the health care system, and its future affordability.

Five overarching issues will shape the future of Medicare. First, Medicare was established to help the elderly and then disabled persons afford medical care. But, many policy analysts have argued that the program inadequately meets the needs of the aged and disabled, which has raised expectations for improvements. Medicare's coverage is less generous than that offered to many younger families and individuals through employer-subsidized insurance. Even with prescription drug coverage, added in 2006, gaps in coverage remain. Second, the economic status of Medicare beneficiaries (both absolutely and compared with younger families) is a critical factor in assessing how the system should change. Perceptions about older persons' well-being have swung sharply since Medicare began in 1966, with once-beleaguered seniors now viewed as very well off. Despite some prosperity, most Medicare beneficiaries have limited resources and cannot afford a substantial increase in health care costs. These two issues, discussed in chapter 1, imply greater pressures for more spending.

Third, demographic changes looming on the horizon—which will swell the ranks of those eligible for benefits and diminish the number of workers financing the system—are beginning to influence the debate even about Medicare's near-term future. The first of the so-called Baby Boom generation will become eligible for Medicare in 2011. Because of increasing life expectancy, this will begin a *permanent* upward shift in the share of the population age 65 and above. Again, these changes add to pressures for growth in Medicare spending. See figure 2.1 for an indication of that demographic growth.

Fourth, what happens in the health care system affects Medicare, and vice versa. In many ways, the problems facing Medicare reflect the broader challenges facing health care in the United States. Health care demands have grown as a share of our national output over time and will likely continue into the future for both Medicare beneficiaries and the entire health care system as new technologies and procedures are developed. It is unrealistic to assume that Medicare can be held to substantially different standards for quality and access to services than the rest of the health care system.

Finally, Medicare's future is tied to the fact that it is a public program. As a result, it is linked to the financing problems facing the federal government during a period of fiscal restraint. So long as budget deficits, which returned after a brief hiatus at the end of the 1990s, continue at the federal level, changes in Medicare will be caught up in the pressure to limit all federal spending. Further, Medicare faces its own financing challenges: a large portion of it is funded by earmarked taxes that do not rise as fast as spending on the program. The claims made about Medicare being "unsustainable" imply that major efforts to limit its size and scope will be necessary.

Public budgeting issues have largely dominated changes in Medicare after 1972 with only one major exception. Attempts to achieve slower program growth have generated ad hoc efforts during the annual federal budget cycles. Over time, these efforts substantially slowed Medicare's rate of growth, culminating in 1997 with substantial cutbacks as part of the Balanced Budget Act. Late in 2003, after years of stalemate over any expansion of Medicare, new legislation passed, adding a substantial new drug benefit. Yet even this legislation reflects the conflicts facing Medicare, including not only increased spending on drugs but further efforts to achieve cost containment. The 2003 expansion could be rolled back in the future; indeed, many members of Congress expressed alarm at the size of projected Medicare spending when the 2006 budget estimates were released. Although the projections had changed very little from when the 2003 legislation passed, the very high spending years of 2014 and 2015 were added to the 10-year estimates, increasing the projected total. The reluctance of politicians and others to even suggest increased revenues complicates the picture.

This chapter continues an overview of Medicare, broadening the issues beyond impacts on beneficiaries. The chapter starts with sources of health care spending growth, then turns to an examination of financing, both for the government as a whole and for Medicare in particular.

MEDICARE AS PART OF THE BROADER HEALTH CARE SYSTEM

The problems driving Medicare costs up are not unique to the public sector. They are found throughout our nation's health care system. The rising costs hit all payers: individuals, businesses, and governments. Although Medicare has led the way in curbing these costs (both in terms of increasing prices and use of services), costs continue to rise.

Prices

During the 1970s, health care prices rose rapidly along with all prices in the economy. In the 1980s, however, the general rise in consumer prices slowed, while health care prices kept growing. After 1980, health care price inflation occurred at rates substantially higher than that for the overall index. Between 1980 and the 2004, all consumer prices net of health care grew 132 percent, while the consumer price index (CPI) for medical care grew 320 percent.[1] Even as medical care prices moderated in the late 1990s, they still remained well above prices for other goods and services.

What caused this inflation in health care prices during the two decades when the growth of other prices slowed substantially? Some economists point to the fact that health care is heavily service oriented, so rising wages translate directly into rising prices. Productivity does not rise much in this sector of the economy, making it difficult to find ways to cut costs per service. This problem exists for all types of service industries, but the differential between medical and other services remains large: 339 percent growth in the price of medical services compared with 165 percent growth for all other services.[2]

Nor is it possible to blame increasing health care prices on strong demand for scarce services. The supply of physicians continued its rapid growth through the 1970s and 1980s. For example, in 1970, the number of active physicians per 10,000 people stood at 15.6. By 1988, the number was 23.3 per 10,000 (National Center for Health Statistics [NCHS] 1991). This greater supply of physicians did not, however, lower their incomes, which rose an average of 8.6 percent per year from 1979 to 1988. Physicians per 10,000 people stood at 27.8 in 2000 (NCHS 2003). Further, hospitals operated at much less than capacity throughout the 1980s, with occupancy rates averaging about 64 percent in 1993 (American Hospital Association [AHA] 1995). In 2001, occupancy rates rose slightly to 66.7 percent (NCHS 2003).

Some of the explanation for rising prices undoubtedly rests with the fact that, for many years, the price structure of the health care industry had not been scrutinized. Users of health care are typically not the payers; usually a "third party," such as an insurance company or the government, pays for the care. Insured people do not have to use price as the basis for their choices about who to see or what to use to the same degree that purchasers of other goods and services do. More important, even when the patient is paying directly, people facing a medical crisis are unlikely to shop around for the least expensive care or to question the need for various services. In short, the market for health care goods and services does not foster price competition. But it is important not to lay all blame on third-party payers. Seniors, who often pay high prices for drugs and lack comprehensive drug insurance, continue to consume nonetheless.

Use of Services

Despite rising prices, use of health care services continues to increase. Indeed, increased use is a larger reason for higher health care spending than price increases. Higher use occurs not just in terms of numbers of visits or treatments but in the type and complexity of health care services used (often referred to as "intensity"). To some extent, this is related to new technology that has given us tools such as computerized tomography (CT) scans, magnetic resonance imagers (MRIs), positron emission tomography scans, and procedures such as endoscopies and arthroscopies. These new sources of health care spending tend to operate as additions to goods and services consumed, rather than as replacements for old technologies or procedures. For example, people may now receive x-rays, CT scans, and MRIs to diagnose a problem, while before only x-rays (and perhaps exploratory surgery) were available. As another example, rather than subjecting a blood sample to one test, 30 or 40 tests can be run per sample.

New tests and procedures that are less invasive and painful improve diagnosis and treatment for many Americans—and increase the frequency of their use. For example, between 1999 and 2002, imaging services paid under the physician fee schedule grew by an average of 9 percent per capita, compared with 3 percent growth for all fee schedule services. And the fastest growing of these services (MRIs, nuclear medicine, and CT) also tend to be the most expensive (MedPAC 2005). Some argue that these services are overused and less advanced tests or fewer alternative tests would suffice. But for the average patient, there is little reason to resist using these tools. Further, not only are physicians paid well for these extra tests, but testing may allow physicians to make diagnoses more quickly. Since low reimbursement discourages doctors from spending large amounts of time with their patients, their reliance on formal tests makes even more sense. So the system works to encourage the development—and use—of new technology.

Surgery and other technical procedures continue to grow, albeit in different settings than in the past. The number of inpatient surgical operations fell by 4.6 percent between 1980 and 1989 (NCHS 1991) largely because of the growth in outpatient surgical procedures occurring in a variety of settings. By 1994, AHA reported that 55.4 percent of total hospital-based surgeries were performed in outpatient departments, compared with just 16.4 percent in 1980 (AHA 1994). And many procedures such as cataract surgery are now done in freestanding surgical centers or even physicians' offices.

Although it is difficult to track surgical procedures since many of them are shifting out of inpatient settings, early work in this area found that inpatient and outpatient surgeries—when combined—continued to rise from 1980 to 1995. Some surgeries switched almost entirely to outpatient settings while others continued to expand in the traditional inpatient setting (Kozak, McCarthy, and Pokras 1999).

Studies on the reasons underlying spending growth for the working age population point to hospital care (both inpatient and outpatient), with two-thirds of that growth attributable to higher use of services (Strunk, Ginsburg, and Gabel 2002). This suggests that inpatient surgeries are becoming increasingly more complex and expensive. For example, while the rate of tonsillectomies dropped dramatically from 1980 to 1993, expensive procedures showed the opposite trend. Cardiac bypass surgery rates for men over the age of 75, for instance, rose from 0.9 per 1,000 in 1980 to 8.7 per 1,000 in 1993 and to 12.2 per 1,000 in 2000 (NCHS 1996, 2002).

The improved success of procedures such as hip replacements and cataract surgery means that outcomes have improved while the risks of surgeries have fallen. In such cases, higher rates of use would certainly be expected and appropriate. The value of these procedures to individuals has increased over time. And lowered risks mean that older or disabled patients are particularly more likely to benefit now. It should not be surprising, then, that costs of care for these groups under Medicare are rising rapidly. In fact, some of the increase in use likely reflects the greater value of such services and that beneficiaries choose to consume more of them. David Cutler (2004) argues persuasively that extending life and enhancing standards of living justify the spending on new technology.

The number of patient contacts with specialists is also on the rise, and the supply of physicians reflects this trend. Between 1975 and 2000, the number of general and family practitioners increased 46 percent, while the number of cardiovascular disease specialists grew 223 percent; orthopedic surgeons, 113 percent; and gastroenterologists, 402 percent (NCHS 2002). These figures also indicate that use is shifting to higher-cost services over time.

The problem, of course, is determining what proportion of the overall increase in use is desirable and what proportion indicates excessive or unnecessary care. Cataract surgery offers a good example. We do not know what share of its explosive growth occurs because people with early cataracts are encouraged to obtain the operation before it is medically appropriate and what share reflects surgeries that truly improve patients' quality of life.

Growth in Medicare Compared with Other Payers

As a public program, Medicare came under pressure to hold the line on costs in the 1980s—earlier than other payers. Many private payers finally began to take note in the 1990s, when price increases slowed as insurers sought discounts from care providers. In the mid-1990s, employers moved their workers into more restrictive managed care plans where use could be actively controlled. Cost growth dropped substantially. But the backlash by consumers against such plans has led to less stringency in recent years—and accelerating premium costs (Strunk et al. 2002). Once again, however, there are concerns about rising prices as service providers have begun to rebel against years of low price growth. For employer-provided insurance, for example, employees are being asked to pay higher premiums, deductibles, and co-payments (Henry J. Kaiser Family Foundation and Health Research and Educational Trust [HRET] 2005).

Compared with private insurance, Medicare mostly held the line on growth in health care costs in the 1980s and 1990s. Figure 2.2 illustrates this comparison and shows cumulative rates of growth in per capita spending in Medicare and private insurance from the national health expenditure accounts on a selected set of services between 1970 and 2000 (Boccuti and Moon 2003). These services—hospital care, physicians and other professional services, and vision and durable medical equipment—are consistently covered by both Medicare and private insurance. Home health and skilled nursing care are excluded since Medicare is more likely to pay for these services. And drugs, which private insurers are more likely to cover, are also excluded from the analysis to create a comparable mix of covered services. Between 1985 and 1992, Medicare had lower rates of growth, often considerably lower, than did private insurance. Growth in private-sector spending also slowed for a time in the mid-1990s. So the data suggest that Medicare is not out of sync with the rest of the health care system.

Figure 2.2. Cumulative Growth in Per Enrollee Payments for Comparable Services, Medicare and Private Insurers, 1970–2000

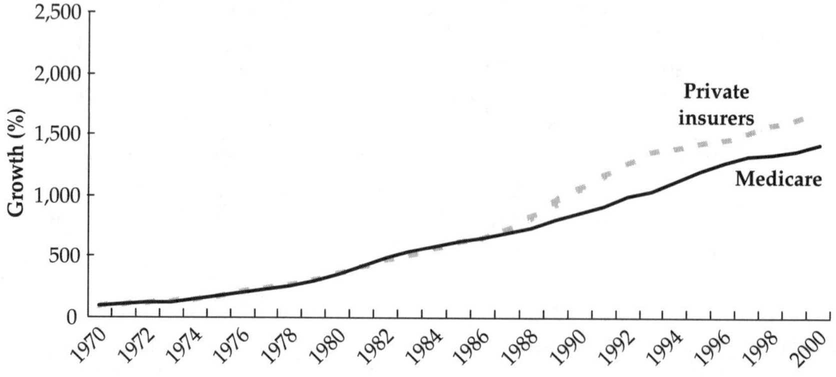

Source: Boccuti and Moon (2003).

Note: Includes hospital care, physician, and clinical services, durable medical equipment, and other professional services.

Indeed, Medicare's patterns in spending growth are very similar to and often below those of private insurance. This is particularly important given factors that could drive up the costs of care for this population relative to others. For example, Medicare's population is aging overall, adding modest pressures for higher spending over time (Moon 1999). Further, as new technology becomes safer and more effective, it is likely to expand faster among more frail populations like aging Medicare beneficiaries.

Critics of this analysis on Medicare growth have pointed out that, during this period, coverage expanded for workers and their families—changes that the data used for this analysis cannot capture well (Antos and King 2003). While such differences may affect the results, much of the expansion in private insurance is associated with the addition of prescription drugs explicitly omitted from this analysis, and lower cost sharing when reliance on managed care increased. These trends reversed by the end of the 1990s as employees' share of premiums and cost sharing increased (Henry J. Kaiser Family Foundation and HRET 2005).

The important lesson from comparing Medicare to other payers is not so much which sector is doing better at holding the line on costs at one point in time, but rather that health care costs tend to change in tandem no matter what the source of payment is. So Medicare cannot successfully hold down costs over the long run if health care spending in general escalates. As stated, the pressures driving costs upward come from all parts of the health care system. Although Medicare commands a substantial share of the health care market, it cannot, by itself, fully control use or prices without creating incredible pressures elsewhere.

When Medicare acts alone, the response by providers can be to "divide and conquer," pitting one part of the system against the other. This constrains what Medicare can accomplish on its own. Broader system reform is needed for any long-term solution to Medicare's "cost problem." Expecting Medicare alone to carry this burden or to operate under a system unlike the rest of health care seems doomed to failure. Alternatively, the recent process of adjusting Medicare incrementally with an awareness of how it compares with the private sector can continue to be used, at least for the time being. For example, payments to physicians were adjusted upwards in 2003 and again in 2004 to correct an error in the formula for setting payments and, more importantly, because of fears that the payments would lag too far behind those in the private sector and would discourage physician participation. The visibility of the Medicare system inevitably invites comparisons with payments and service use elsewhere.

MEDICARE AS PART OF THE FEDERAL BUDGET

Medicare's absolute size and rate of growth cause it to stand out from most other domestic programs in the federal budget. Further, because tax dollars fund Medicare in an era of antitax sentiment, it gets more scrutiny than health expenditures financed directly by individuals or businesses. In the view of many policymakers during the 1990s, Medicare was crowding out expenditures on other domestic programs and standing in the way of controlling growth in federal expenditures. Such critics often argue that Americans will only accept a certain level of public spending, so if Medicare grows rapidly, it hurts other programs, even if it has its own revenue source. This makes it a target.

The portion of the federal budget devoted to health care expanded since 1965, when Medicare was enacted. Critics pointed out early on that Medicare spending was likely to grow rapidly, and it did. For example, in 1970, spending on Medicare totaled $6.8 billion, about 3.5 percent of the total federal budget (figure 2.3). Ten years later, that share more than doubled as Medicare accounted for 8.6 percent of the federal budget and about $107 billion in outlays in 1980 (U.S. Congress, Committee on Ways and Means 1991). By 2004, the share had grown to 13 percent of the budget (U.S. Congressional Budget Office 2004).

Because Medicare is such a large component of the federal budget, it receives particular scrutiny as a potential source of budget savings. And when it has grown much faster than other budget components, substantial "savings" can be achieved by slowing the rate of spending

Figure 2.3. Medicare as a Share of the Federal Budget

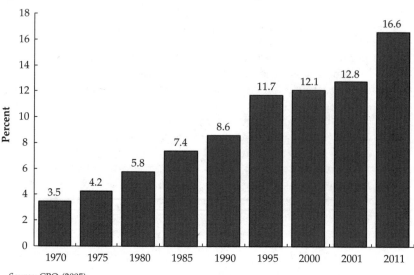

Source: CBO (2005).

growth. Many of the changes made under the Balanced Budget Act of 1997 were of a different order of magnitude, however, and generated a slowdown well beyond what was originally anticipated. In fact, aggregate spending on Medicare declined in 1999 while the number of enrollees increased. Spending on some services remained lower than 1998 levels for a number of years. After 2001, Medicare again grew rapidly and captured policymakers' attention just as overall budget deficits returned with a vengeance.

Adding to budgetary pressures, many Americans view Medicare with the same skepticism with which they view public programs and government spending in general. Because it is a government program, Medicare is automatically labeled bureaucratic and wasteful. As noted, however, the private sector has not generally been more successful in curbing the growth in health care spending. Further, evidence suggests that some problems arise more from spending too little on administration rather than too much. For example, complaints about poor services and Medicare's complexity result in part from tight budgets for processing claims. Compared with the private insurance sector, the Centers for Medicare and Medicaid Services (CMS, the new name for the Health Care Financing Administration) administrative costs for running the Medicare program are quite low, totaling only about 2 to 3 percent of benefit payments, compared with larger proportional amounts—around 6 to 15 percent—for private insurers (Congressional Research Service 1989), and more than 20 percent for Medigap (GAO 2001).

MEASURING MEDICARE'S FINANCIAL HEALTH

In addition to broad federal budget issues, financing Medicare requires individual attention. Medicare is currently financed in a variety of ways. Part A relies mainly on payroll taxes with a modest contribution from income taxes on Social Security benefits. Part B is financed by enrollee premiums set at 25 percent of the costs of Part B benefits for elderly beneficiaries, and by general revenue contributions sufficient to cover the remaining costs. Part D will use essentially the same financing structure as Part B.

Medicare's financial health can be viewed from several perspectives. The appropriate question over time is whether, *as a society*, we can afford to support Medicare. That is, are health care costs for the elderly and disabled beneficiaries likely to be so high that some people will need to go without care? And how should that be balanced against health care priorities across all age groups and compared with other spending? If policymakers examine only current revenue burdens and the potential for greater federal revenue contributions in the future, then limiting government spending seems to "solve" the problem. But since people need to get care somewhere, if the burdens are shifted onto beneficiaries and their families, *society* will be no better off. In that case, the issue essentially becomes one of *who* should pay. Raising revenues dedicated to the Part A Trust Fund, for example, also could "solve" the problem. It is important to look carefully at the claims made on Medicare's financial status and recognize that both spending and financing issues are at stake.

Solvency Measures

The first and most commonly cited solvency measure is the date of exhaustion of the Part A Trust Fund.[3] This is one of several basic measures that have traditionally been reported in the Medicare Board of Trustees annual reports on Medicare's financial outlook (Boards of Trustees 2005). Critics of Medicare have pointed to the solvency of the Part A Trust Fund as an indicator of affordability, treating the Part A Trust Fund as establishing a limit on what can be spent on Part A. A number of improvements in the solvency measure used to examine Medicare have been proposed, several of which are examined below.

Part A Trust Fund Solvency. The Part A Trust Fund was designed to ensure that the designated payroll tax contribution would be used specifically for Part A–Hospital Insurance (HI) spending. As dedicated revenues, payroll and other revenue sources that exceed the amount necessary to cover Part A benefits go into the trust fund and collect interest. When the trust fund forecasts indicate a declining balance, this warns of the need for adjusting either revenue contributions or spending.[4]

Projections of the Medicare Part A Trust Fund indicate that it will maintain a positive balance through 2020 (Board of Trustees 2005). Since 2001, the date of projected insolvency has moved up, but still remains further into the future than it has been over most of Medicare's history (figure 2.4). The trust fund balance in 2004 was $269 billion or 158 percent of annual Part A expenditures. It is expected to grow to $334 billion in 2011 and then decline over time as a share of Part A spending. Certainly this signals a need for change.

However, this measure ignores Part B issues and so does not take into account the full size of the Medicare program. But since automatic infusions of general revenue keep Part B's trust fund in balance and funding for the two parts are kept separate by law, a "solvency" measure is difficult to devise for Medicare as a whole.

Critics also argue that the trust fund is merely an accounting fiction and that the assets now reported are not "real." This is because the dollars that have come into the Treasury above what is needed to pay Part A benefits are used for other purposes while the fund holds Treasury securities and earns interest on them. However, just like other

Figure 2.4. Number of Years Before HI Trust Fund Projected to Be Exhausted

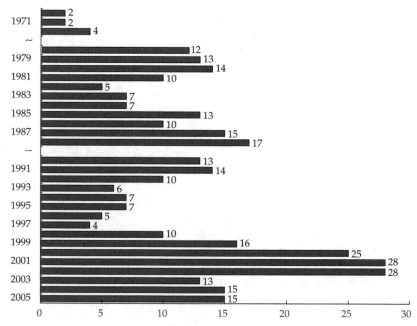

Sources: Congressional Research Service (1995) and Board of Trustees (2005).
~ data not available for 1973–1977 and 1989.

federal bondholders, Medicare should be able to count on the promises made when the bonds were issued—that is, that they would be honored in later years when Part A revenues are not sufficient to cover spending. In this sense, the bonds Medicare holds are no different from other Treasury securities that are treated in the marketplace as largely "without risk." Although the dollars are real, there is a legitimate question of whether the surplus funds are used productively.[5]

An Alternative Solvency Measure. An alternative measure of Medicare's financial health proposed by some budget analysts in recent years paints an even direr picture of Medicare's future. This "new" measure of solvency—put forth by the Bush administration in its fiscal year (FY) 2003 and 2004 budgets and by the Congressional Budget Office in its January 2002 Medicare baseline—combines all Part A and B spending but only shows *part* of the revenue sources as defined by current law. While a unified measure of solvency could be advantageous in taking into account both portions of Medicare spending, this approach provides an unbalanced comparison of spending and revenues over time. This approach to describing Medicare's financial outlook omits general revenue sources entirely from the presentation of Medicare revenues and includes only "dedicated" revenues (payroll taxes and premiums) in comparisons of future projected revenues and costs. This approach is at variance with current law by ignoring contributions from general revenues as a source of Medicare funding, even though these revenues have been a part of the program since its inception.

As figure 2.5 shows, this gives the appearance of a substantially lower revenue stream for Medicare over time. In its FY 2003 budget, the administration referred to the program as being "in deficit" because dedicated taxes (mainly payroll tax revenues and premiums) were insufficient to cover spending in that year. But this is a misrepresentation because general revenue contributions (an explicitly designated source of funding under current law) are ignored.[6] This is comparable to arguing that defense spending is fully in deficit because it relies entirely on general revenue funding.

Affordability Measures

Assessing affordability on the basis of the solvency of the Part A Trust Fund is analogous to individuals arguing that they cannot pay all their bills because the balance in *one* of their checking accounts is too low. Affordability is a broader issue that turns on whether we as a society *can* support Medicare into the future. The Medicare Trustees' annual report offers two broader measures of affordability, although each are

Figure 2.5. Medicare Solvency Issues Raised by Counting only Dedicated Revenues

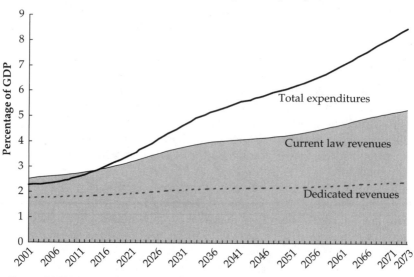

Sources: OASDI (2001) and Medicare Trustees Reports (various years).

limited in scope (Boards of Trustees 2005). Finally, a new third measure offered here proposes a more comprehensive way to examine afford-ability.

The Worker-to-Beneficiary Ratio. The ratio of workers contributing to Medicare at any point in time compared with the number of benefi-ciaries shows that, given the aging of society, the number of younger persons relative to older ones will decline in the future. This declining ratio of workers to retirees indicates that each worker will have to bear a larger share of the cost of providing payroll tax–financed Medicare benefits.

The numbers are quite dramatic (figure 2.6). Between 2000 and 2035 (several years beyond when most Baby Boomers will have become eligible for Medicare),[7] the ratio of workers to beneficiaries will fall from 3.90 to 2.21. This change represents a 43 percent decline in the ratio through 2035. Indeed, this is one statistic commonly cited by those who claim the program is "unsustainable." It does signal the need for more revenues per worker—a legitimate issue for debate. However, it fails to assess the level of burden relative to each future worker's ability to pay, ignoring any improvement in the economic circumstances of workers over time due to per capita economic growth.

Medicare Spending as a Share of GDP. A second measure, which has long been included in the annual reports but is now getting more attention, is the sum of Part A and B spending as a share of GDP. In 2000, Medicare's total share was 2.3 percent and is projected to rise to

Figure 2.6. Ratio of Workers to Medicare Beneficiaries (2000–2035)

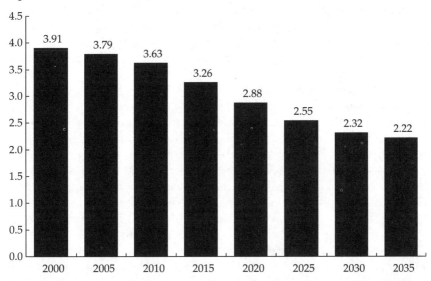

Source: American Institutes for Research analysis of 2005 OASDI and Medicare Trustees Reports.

5.0 percent in 2030 for Parts A and B and to 6.8 percent when prescription drugs are included (see figure 2.1). This represents nearly a tripling of the GDP share. This increase reflects the fact that health care costs per capita are expected to continue rising, and the number of people covered will double over that period.

This measure (Medicare spending as a share of GDP) also puts potential costs into the context of U.S. aggregate production and offers more information than the worker-to-retiree ratio. In addition, since both Parts A and B are included in the measure, it provides a broader look into the future than when only Part A solvency is examined. It is not a very intuitive measure, however, as there is no natural benchmark for what an appropriate share would be, particularly as the share of the population covered by Medicare rises over time. In addition, it may not be as helpful in the debate on Medicare's future because it does not consider how well off we will be as a society as GDP grows. Some goods and services, like health care, may appropriately grow as a share of GDP in response to higher living standards.

A More Comprehensive Measure of Affordability. Another way to look at affordability is to focus not on the *number* of workers that contribute to payroll and income taxes, nor on aggregate GDP, but instead on how the Medicare per capita burden will affect workers over time. While the share of the pie (GDP) that goes to Medicare is likely to increase, if the pie (on a per capita basis) also increases, then an increasing share is less of a burden.[8] If the future leads to greater national well-being, additional resource sharing would be affordable. So another way to examine affordability is to focus on whether taxpayers in the future will be better off even *after* they pay higher amounts for Medicare. Such a measure examines whether, as a society, we can *afford* such care for this population.

The measure begins with computing GDP per worker over time, which measures the nation's output of goods and services divided across the working population (table 2.1). This provides the base for assessing Medicare's burden on workers, who pay the bulk of support for the program. Per-worker GDP—even after adjusting for inflation—rises substantially from $74,914 per worker in 2005 to over $124,421 in 2035 (in 2004 dollars).[9] This is an increase of 66.1 percent in per worker GDP, a substantial increase in financial well-being.

What about Medicare's costs over this period? The burdens from Medicare spending on each worker are projected to rise at a faster rate than per-capita GDP because both numbers of beneficiaries and their inflation-adjusted spending will rise over time. But because per-worker GDP is a much larger dollar amount than Medicare burdens, the reduction in well-being that this will entail for workers is modest.

To calculate the per-worker burden from Medicare, several adjustments are necessary. First, each worker will bear an increasing share of Medicare over time because of the change in the ratio of workers to retirees. Further, per-capita Medicare costs are expected to rise faster than GDP by 2035, also increasing the real dollar burden on workers. But workers do not bear all of Medicare's costs. Costs are adjusted downward by projected beneficiary contributions. The Part B and D premiums are one financing source netted out of the total. In addition, beneficiaries make further contributions because some of the taxation of Social Security benefits goes into Part A, and older and disabled persons also pay income taxes that help support Parts B and D. So those costs also need to be netted out when calculating per-worker burden.

The resulting real per-worker burden estimates range from $1,906 in 2005 to $5,567 in 2035 (in 2004 dollars) based on Medicare spending *before* adding in the costs of prescription drugs. The burden in 2035 rises to $7,303 per worker when the drug benefit is included. The first column in table 2.1 indicates per-worker GDP in inflation-adjusted dollars, and the third column indicates how much of per-worker GDP remains after accounting for the Medicare burden. From 2005 to 2035, the increase in net (after subtracting Medicare minus its drug benefit) per-worker resources would be 60.0 percent, compared with the 66.1 percent increase in per-worker GDP. When the cost of the new drug burden is added, the growth in per-worker GDP falls to 57.2 percent. That is, workers would still be substantially better off than today, even

Table 2.1. GDP Per Capita for Workers Adjusted for Projected Medicare Burdens (2004$)

Year	Per capita GDP	Per capita GDP minus Medicare burden (Parts A and B only)	Per capita GDP minus Medicare burden (Parts A, B, and D)
2005	74,914	73,035	72,934
2010	80,272	78,133	77,637
2015	85,555	83,019	82,334
2020	90,924	87,775	86,835
2025	96,757	92,833	91,603
2030	103,008	98,186	96,689
2035	109,710	103,931	102,189
2040	116,846	110,104	108,129

Source: Author's calculations based on Boards of Trustees (2005).
GDP = gross domestic product

after paying the full projected costs of Medicare with the prescription drug benefit.[10]

The pie will indeed have gotten larger. There will, of course, be other demands on these resources, but this approach puts demands from Medicare into a broader perspective. This measure for examining affordability takes Parts A, B, and D into account, and puts the issue of the burdens into a per-worker context that is likely to be more meaningful to individuals looking into the future.

This more comprehensive measure of net per-worker output also suggests that, as a society, we will be able to afford Medicare without an inordinate burden on workers or taxpayers once even modest estimates of productivity growth over time are taken into account. However, tax rates would have to rise to pay for such benefits. The challenge will be for society to decide whether it is *willing* to pay some or all of these costs.

RETHINKING MEDICARE POLICY

Will the pressures for change in Medicare result in program growth or contraction? The rest of this book has two goals: to describe and analyze Medicare's growth and development and to assess future options for change. Medicare rapidly enrolled persons age 65 and over in 1966, and persons with disabilities in 1974, offering them access to mainstream medical care. But doing so led to a demand for services that helped create rapid growth in federal outlays. Much of Medicare's recent history has involved efforts to hold the line on cost growth. And although its growth has continued, Medicare has been relatively successful at cost containment, with innovations in hospital and physician payment that have led the way for the private sector.

But despite its successes in cost containment, Medicare leaves many of its critics unsatisfied. Further reductions in spending will be sought by those concerned with the "bloated" size of the program, and some of those cuts are bound to occur in an area where we have already seen considerable change: payments to health care providers. Additional pressures will be levied on beneficiaries to pay more. Even in the absence of changes to save costs, Medicare cost sharing is due for reexamination. It is too high in some areas, too low in others, and was never designed to appropriately influence incentives to consume health care services.

Some criticism of Medicare results in calls for more substantive policy change. Incremental increases in premiums, cost sharing, and provider payments will not satisfy those who believe the program should be severely scaled back. In that case, more dramatic realignments would be required. Calls for decentralizing the program and relying on the private sector to oversee a restructuring have been made for over a decade. However, the evidence to support the effectiveness of such a change has, if anything, weakened over time.

Counterbalancing these proposals are suggestions for expanding Medicare—adding better catastrophic protection, further expanding coverage of prescription drugs, or, most dramatically, bringing long-term care under Medicare's umbrella. Willingness to share the burdens of health care gets higher marks from the general public than from policymakers (Oberlander 2003). At this juncture, it is difficult to project what the future holds for Medicare.

3

HOW MEDICARE HAS CHANGED: COVERAGE AND BENEFIT PAYMENTS

M edicare—a program that has had an enormous impact on those it serves—celebrated its 40th birthday in 2005. But over the years, many changes have occurred, mainly by adding new beneficiaries and by facing substantial challenges aimed at reducing the growth in spending on the program.

BEFORE MEDICARE

When Medicare passed on July 28, 1965, its overriding goal was to provide mainstream health care for Americans age 65 and older. At the time, the health system underserved the elderly, largely because many could not afford to obtain care. Insurance coverage was rarely part of retirement benefits, and private insurance companies were reluctant to sell coverage to older persons even when seniors could afford it.

In the early 1960s, older Americans were disproportionately poor compared with the rest of the population. The 1962 poverty rate for elderly families was 47 percent, as opposed to 13 percent for families headed by someone age 25 to 54 (Council of Economic Advisors 1964). Many older persons had incomes just above the official poverty level and could not afford even modest insurance, despite lower health insurance costs than now.

Some public support for low-income older Americans was available, primarily in the form of Medical Assistance to the Aged (MAA).[1] This legislation was originally part of the Kerr-Mills bill, passed in 1960. MAA required a means test, but it was not restricted to persons receiving public assistance. Rather, it was a federal and state matching program, and states were able to set eligibility limits wherever they wished. Although MAA can be viewed as a precursor to Medicare and Medicaid, it was always a very limited program. In 1963, only 148,000 elderly persons received MAA, compared with Medicare's enrollment of 19 million persons by 1967 (Newman 1972). In 1965, MAA provided $523 million in medical benefits to the elderly.[2] In its first two years of existence, Medicare spending on the elderly poor grew to $2.1 billion— four times greater than MAA's level in 1965 (Plotnick and Skidmore 1976).

For higher-income elderly persons, the story was mixed. About half of all seniors had health insurance (Andersen, Lion, and Anderson 1976; Davis and Schoen 1978). Coverage could be obtained through former employers and from groups such as the American Association of Retired Persons (AARP). But for some, health insurance was not merely an issue of affordability; it was one of availability at any price. Private insurers had shown a reluctance to cover the elderly. Although many older Americans lacked health care, even in 1965 this was not a homogeneous group.

In contrast, coverage of workers through their employers became increasingly common in the 1950s, underscoring discrepancies between elderly and nonelderly access to care. Although health insurance was a relative oddity at the end of World War II, it quickly became an important benefit for many workers (Starr 1982). By 1960, the United States was separating into two camps: the health care haves and have-nots. The elderly contained a disproportionate share of the have-nots.

THE GENESIS OF MEDICARE

President Lyndon Johnson signed Medicare into law on July 30, 1965, in a ceremony in Independence, Missouri, honoring the important role that President Harry Truman had played in the national health insurance debate since World War II. Truman never saw passage of a national health care program during his presidency, but his advocacy was credited with starting the process. Over time, the debate shifted to ensuring coverage for the elderly as the most vulnerable and deserving subgroup of the population. The election of President Johnson in 1964 set the stage for Medicare's passage.

Covering senior citizens was a logical starting point for government action. The 1965 Medicare legislation was one of the major accomplishments of President Johnson's Great Society. However, Medicare had its origins in much earlier proposals. The Roosevelt administration studied the issue and, in 1943, Senators Robert Wagner, James Murray, and John Dingall, Sr., introduced a bill that created a comprehensive national health insurance system paid for with payroll taxes (Starr 1982). President Truman also mounted a major effort in the late 1940s when he called for a national program (Marmor 1970).

Evolution of the Legislation

Public provision of health insurance was not popular during the administration of Dwight Eisenhower; employer-provided insurance continued to expand, and health care costs remained low. Nonetheless, the long history of support for public health insurance contains many Republican as well as Democratic supporters. For example, Republican Earl Warren, while governor of California, proposed compulsory health insurance for the state in 1945 (Somers and Somers 1967). However, Republican opposition, coupled with the vociferous opposition of the American Medical Association (AMA), doomed this and all other related national legislative initiatives through the 1950s.

The issue never died, however. A number of influential leaders in the field of social insurance, including Robert Ball, I. S. Falk, Wilbur Cohen, and American Federation of Labor leader Nelson Cruikshank developed a bill that was introduced by Congressman Aime Forand of Rhode Island in 1957. Well-publicized hearings were held, and the bill, though failing to pass, rallied Democrats to push their proposals in health (Campion 1984; Myers 1970). In 1959, President Eisenhower's secretary of Health, Education, and Welfare, Arthur Flemming, released a report on options for providing hospital insurance to Social Security beneficiaries.

After supporting such legislation in the U.S. Senate, John F. Kennedy pledged in his presidential campaign to offer legislation for health insurance for the elderly. Within a month of taking office, President Kennedy delivered to Congress a message calling for such legislation. Congressman Cecil King of California and Senator Clinton Anderson of New Mexico introduced bills that became the focus of debate throughout the early 1960s (Marmor 1970).

But President Kennedy was unable to pass health care coverage for the elderly. Not until after his assassination did a more sympathetic environment for his proposals develop. After the 1964 elections created a lopsided victory for the Democrats, President Johnson pushed Medicare and other Great Society legislation through Congress. With significant help from organized labor, which supported the legislation through its National Council of Senior Citizens, Medicare finally passed.

Even these efforts might not have prevailed without the "conversion" of Congressman Wilbur Mills. As the influential chairman of the House Ways and Means Committee, Mills was in a position to stop any legislation for health insurance. At first, Mills was not inclined to move; he had counted noses and did not have enough support in the House to pass the legislation. Mills was not a legislator who took on lost causes. But with President Johnson's landslide victory, some health care legislation seemed inevitable, so Mills took up the cause to control the outcome. Suspense then centered on what shape the plan would take.

Sensing that stonewalling was unlikely to work, opponents began to develop alternatives. For example, the AMA, believing that the best it could achieve was to limit eligibility, lobbied relentlessly to restrict Medicare to the elderly poor. The AMA favored the Kerr-Mills Medical Assistance to the Aged approach (Derthick 1979), which would limit the size and influence of the public plan, effectively blocking it from becoming a mainstream health care program. Republicans embraced this AMA alternative.

Supporters of Medicare viewed a means-tested approach as dangerous. One of the reasons for focusing first on the elderly had been to avoid creating a means-tested health care program. The precursor means-tested programs had remained very limited in scope. Universal coverage offered the major political advantage of promising benefits for all—an approach that had proven popular with Social Security. Supporters felt this was crucial for Medicare as well.

The leaders stressed social insurance—that is, universal coverage financed by broad-based taxes—and they went to considerable lengths to assert that all, or nearly all, the elderly had incomes too low to afford insurance (Marmor 1970). This was certainly an overstatement, but the claim was made to argue that it would not be worthwhile to means–test (i.e., restrict benefits to persons with low incomes and other resources) the benefits. The debate over means testing assumed a broad significance since both sides recognized that this issue would dramatically affect the public's perception of the plan and influence future policy moves in health care.

The breadth of services this new health plan would cover also became an issue. The King-Anderson bill, although making all the elderly eligible for benefits, was limited to hospital insurance. Proponents of social insurance saw the bill as a first step. Further benefits could be added later if the public accepted the concept of national insurance for hospital services for one portion of the population. Supporters worried about the costs of the initial undertaking, so they proceeded cautiously and kept it limited to hospital services.

Advocates of expanding coverage further came from both sides of the debate. Liberal enthusiasts wanted fully comprehensive care. For example, the Forand bill introduced in 1957 was more inclusive, and other advocates went further with their proposals. Ironically, the major proponents of broader coverage were the conservatives. The AMA and Republican strategy was to argue that it was better to cover the poor comprehensively than to serve everyone partially. Consequently, their alternative bill was much more inclusive in terms of covered services than the Democratic proposal.

Together, the eligibility and coverage issues could have stalemated the entire process. For months, the different parties wrangled and threatened to divide the interest groups lining up for and against various approaches. The AMA and the unions expended enormous sums to influence both public opinion and Congress. In retrospect, the elderly interest groups, often cited as key players today, laid low during these debates. Only the newly created National Council of Senior Citizens, which was effectively a subsidiary of the American Federation of Labor–Congress of Industrial Organizations (AFL-CIO), was prominent. The AARP, which already had a membership of more than 10 million people in 1964, kept a conspicuously low profile. In 1959, the AARP testified for a public–private partnership in which the Social Security system would serve only as a premium-collecting entity to help foster private insurance, such as its own Colonial Penn policies. Note that none of the major histories of Medicare tout significant roles for the AARP (Davis and Schoen 1978; Marmor 1970; Myers 1970; Skidmore 1970: Somers and Somers 1967). The important players in later policy changes in Medicare are quite different from those who led the first charge.

Medicare's Initial Years

The Medicare bill that emerged stunned all observers. The final package Mills put together went beyond what either side had proposed. Mills's solution to the impasse over the competing approaches was to establish two programs: Medicare and Medicaid. Medicare would cover all those 65 and over and would be divided into two parts: Part A, Hospital Insurance (plus skilled nursing care), and Part B, Supplementary Medical Insurance, a voluntary but subsidized insurance plan covering physician services. Medicaid would be targeted to low-income persons of all ages who were participating in other welfare programs.[3] That is, for the elderly, it would fill the gaps created by cost sharing or coverage limitations.

The basic structure of the Medicare program, with its large variety of benefits and patchwork of limitations and definitions, resulted from the negotiations between the House and the Senate. In particular, Senator Russell Long insisted on some changes to add further catastrophic protections,[4] and Part B developed from a proposal from Congressman John Byrnes (R-WI) (Myers 1970). The outcome was a complicated structure of hospital benefits with coinsurance days and lifetime reserve days (defined in appendix A). The legislation as passed in July 1965 had a starting date of July 1, 1966 (then the beginning of the federal fiscal year). From that date on, Medicare and Medicaid fundamentally transformed the shape of American health care. Rather than sinking Medicare, the AMA's opposition not only helped create Medicaid but inadvertently fostered an expanded scope of Medicare benefits (Marmor 1970).

The rules established to govern Medicare did little to disrupt or change the way health care was practiced or financed in the United States. Claims processing was structured to resemble that found in the private sector and was handled by private contractors. And Medicare statutes specifically ensured free choice of provider and no interference in the routine practice of medicine. Payment rates were also designed to resemble those in the private sector, both in the mechanics and level of payment. Physicians' and other providers' groups that participated in the new program at least would not be put at a disadvantage.

But even though the early emphasis was on ensuring that individuals would be covered and included in mainstream medical care, no one was sure that the AMA would not get the last laugh. Their ominous warnings about dangerous moves to socialized medicine carried the implicit threat that physicians might shun patients who were enrolled in either of these new programs. Indeed, in the *New York Times* (August 12, 1965), the Association of American Physicians and Surgeons called for a boycott of Medicare.

But the new programs proved remarkably successful from the beginning. Large numbers of the elderly enrolled, and the use of services expanded rapidly. There was no noticeable boycott by health care providers. By May 31, 1966, 17.6 million elderly persons had enrolled in the optional Part B plan—out of approximately 19 million who were eligible. And in the first three years of Medicare, about 100,000 eligible enrollees were admitted to hospitals each week (Myers 1970). Medicare led to a major increase in the elderly's use of medical care. Hospital discharges averaged 190 per 1,000 elderly persons in 1964 and 350 per 1,000 by 1973, for example, with most of the change occurring in the early years (Davis and Schoen 1978).[5] The proportion of the elderly using physician services jumped from 68 to 76 percent between 1963 and 1970 (Andersen et al. 1973).

Initially, everyone over the age of 65 was eligible. The legislation stressed access to care, without requiring a period of payroll tax contributions to achieve eligibility. This ensured a considerable windfall to persons who reached age 65 before 1968. After grandfathering in the elderly, Medicare eligibility was limited to persons both over the age of 65 and entitled to Social Security benefits, either as workers or dependents.

The payroll contributions that persons in their late 50s and early 60s made into the Medicare trust fund in those early years did not nearly compensate for the costs of health care they received. Further, as costs of health care in general escalated in the 1970s, Medicare spending grew much faster than anticipated, and the "windfalls" to beneficiaries did not decline as anticipated after the first wave of blanket eligibility. The rising costs of health care took everyone by surprise—and the phenomenon was not limited to Medicare.

Health Care Financing Administration actuaries estimated that an elderly individual with average covered earnings retiring in 1982 would have paid in $2,200 and would have had $31,500 in expected future lifetime benefits—a ratio of 14.3 to 1 (U.S. Congressional Budget Office 1983). This was higher than expected because health care costs had risen so rapidly. Over time, however, the ratio did improve. A study in 1991 found that the contribution for an average worker retiring in that year would total $15,416 but that expected lifetime benefits would be $44,368—a ratio of 2.9 to 1 (Christensen 1992). Throughout the history of Medicare, workers' contributions to the system have been less than the returns in benefit payments, although the ratio of benefits to contributions has declined.[6]

Since Medicare's beginning, three types of changes have been debated and sometimes adopted:

- eligibility expansions;
- changes in payments to and controls on providers; and
- benefit expansions.

Eligibility expansions came first with the 1972 Social Security Amendments and with smaller adjustments later. Legislation from the late 1970s through the 1990s often sought to rein in the costs of Medicare. The most important set of changes occurred under the Balanced Budget Act of 1997 (BBA) which reduced spending on the program by more than any of the earlier efforts to limit Medicare's growth. There have been few benefit expansions with the exceptions of the Medicare Catastrophic Coverage Act, passed (in 1988) and then repealed in 1989, and

the recent Medicare Prescription Drug, Improvement, and Modernization Act of 2003. Chapter 4 will discuss benefit expansions and these
acts in more detail.

EXPANSION IN ELIGIBILITY

Most of the initial attention on Medicare centered on whether to make
other groups eligible for the program. In fact, as mentioned earlier,
many Medicare supporters thought its passage was a first step toward
universal insurance coverage. In the Social Security program, coverage
for the disabled was added in 1956 and expanded in 1960 (U.S. Social
Security Administration 2004). Adding the disabled Social Security
recipients represented a logical next step for Medicare.

The 1972 Social Security Amendments

Ultimately, inclusion of disabled persons under Medicare came in 1972
as part of the sweeping Social Security amendments that substantially
increased the commitments of all aspects of the program.[7] The disability
expansion was added by Congress, however, and was not part of
the proposal that President Richard Nixon submitted to the Congress
(Derthick 1979).

Like the calls for covering the elderly, there had been a considerable
history of calls for including disabled individuals in Medicare. The
1963–64 Advisory Council on Social Security had recommended coverage for this group. And although disabled persons were left out of the
1965 legislation, the Johnson administration proposed including them
in 1967. Instead, a new advisory commission was set up and, in 1968,
again recommended coverage. This commission advocated covering
all disabled beneficiaries and insured workers who had been disabled
for three months, resulting in a shorter waiting period than that for cash
benefits (Myers 1970). This would not be part of the final amendments.

One concession to holding down costs for disabled persons was to
limit Medicare eligibility to persons with disabilities who had been
receiving Social Security for at least two years. This meant that workers
not only had to qualify as permanently and totally disabled (a condition
for Social Security benefits, including a five-month waiting period),
but they had to have stayed on the rolls for 24 months. Generally,
eligibility for Social Security disability requires the worker to have paid
payroll taxes for 20 out of the last 40 quarters (U.S. Social Security
Administration 1991).[8]

A last-minute addition created coverage for persons with end-stage
renal disease (ESRD). This was not a new issue to Congress; many bills

had previously been offered to provide for treatment of ESRD, partly in response to the publicity war waged over the fact that this was a treatable disease but average citizens could not afford the treatment (Rettig 1982). Long-term kidney failure is fatal without dialysis or a kidney transplant. Waiting lists and care rationing highlighted a problem where patients were dying not because there was no effective treatment but because of budget constraints and the resulting limited supply of dialysis machines.

ESRD coverage was added by an amendment offered in the Senate at the end of the floor debate, was then included in the conference report with less than 10 minutes of discussion, and hence became part of the final law (Rettig 1976). This lack of consideration did not indicate consensus regarding the inclusion of ESRD patients. Indeed, the creation of a category of patients eligible for Medicare based solely on a particular condition caused many to worry that a "disease-of-the-month" approach might be adopted gradually, making more and more people eligible for coverage.[9] Indeed, the numbers of kidney dialysis patients increased more rapidly than many expected. By 2004, their number had grown to 200,000 at an average annual cost of about $23,000 per beneficiary (Boards of Trustees 2004). These figures reflect the number of persons becoming eligible for benefits and, more importantly, the longevity these treatments provide.

The two groups the 1972 amendments added to Medicare's rolls expanded the number of beneficiaries 10 percent and raised the costs of the program even more since, on average, disabled persons were initially more expensive to cover than the elderly (U.S. Congress, Committee on Ways and Means 1992). Figure 3.1 tracks the rate of growth in Medicare beneficiaries over time and shows the impact of these new beneficiaries.

Although ESRD was a highly visible and expensive disease, it was not the only expensive, deadly disease. But coverage for only one other disease has been specifically added—and even then in a more limited way—perhaps due to the high cost of covering ESRD patients over the past 20 years. In 2000, persons receiving Social Security disability who had amyotrophic lateral sclerosis (ALS, or Lou Gehrig's disease) were made eligible for Medicare with no waiting period.[10]

Other Changes in Access

Medicare has not been extended to any other broad group since 1972; indeed, most changes affecting coverage have been fine-tuning efforts at the margins. So far, Medicare has not served as the first step toward national health insurance. After serious debate in the 1970s, that issue

Figure 3.1. Annual Percentage Change in Number of Medicare Enrollees, CY 1967–2004

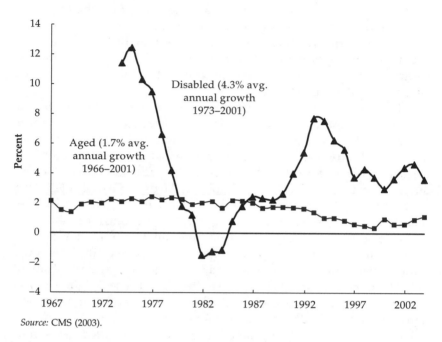

Source: CMS (2003).

was set aside until the late 1980s.[11] Changes after 1972—even in eligibility—largely emphasized cost containment.

Take the case of Medicare "expansion" to all federal workers, passed as part of the Tax Equity and Fiscal Responsibility Act (TEFRA) of 1982 (U.S. Congress, Committee on Ways and Means 1985). Initially, Medicare coverage was not offered to federal workers since they had their own health care system. In practice, however, many federal workers became eligible for Medicare through other means. In some cases, their spouses were eligible and they became entitled by being elderly dependents of covered workers. Many federal workers shifted between the private and the public sectors over their working lives. Consequently, they might have contributed little but qualified for a minimal Social Security check and the full range of Medicare benefits. This "expansion" to new federal workers was actually a budget-reduction effort requiring all such workers to pay the Medicare portion of the FICA tax for their working lives. A similar expansion in 1986 included all newly hired state and local workers.

Other budget-reducing legislation in 1982 limited eligibility for the working elderly (age 65 to 69). This legislation required Medicare to be the "secondary payer" for employed persons who have access to employer-provided health insurance: private insurance was made responsible for paying most of an individual's health care bills, while Medicare pays only for services not otherwise covered. This effectively shifted costs onto employers. This change sought to reduce federal Medicare spending without lowering insurance coverage for beneficiaries. These workers were guaranteed at least all the benefits Medicare offered. The only question was who pays for that coverage. This provision was later extended to all Medicare beneficiaries.

During the 1980s, the Reagan administration moved to restrict disability beneficiaries' eligibility by enforcing tougher standards under Social Security. Restricting access to the cash-benefit program also reduced the number of eligible individuals. These efforts substantially slowed the rate of growth in the number of new disability beneficiaries during the 1980s (see figure 3.1). From 1975 to 1981, growth in disability beneficiaries averaged 5.6 percent per year. However, this growth almost came to a standstill between 1981 and 1986 and has since grown only slightly. Over the entire 1981 to 1989 period, it averaged just 0.7 percent annually (U.S. Congress, Committee on Ways and Means 1991). From 1990 to 2002, the number of disability enrollees grew from 3.3 million to 5.8 million—yielding growth averaging 4.8 percent per year (CMS 2004a).[12] This growth is expected to slow again in the future.

The changes since 1972 have been limited and reflect the retrenchment from expanding access at the beginning of the program. No substantial cuts have occurred in the two major groups Medicare covers, although later chapters will address several proposals for cuts that have received attention.

CONTAINING COSTS IN FEE-FOR-SERVICE MEDICARE

Not long after enactment, Medicare began to be viewed with alarm—not because of its failure but because of its success. The rapid initial growth in the cost of the program showed how quickly the system could fulfill its goal of offering mainstream medical care to older persons. The share of seniors using services expanded from 53 percent in 1975 to 64 percent in 1985 (CMS 2004a). The addition of disabled and ESRD patients in 1972 increased program costs substantially.

It is not surprising, then, that the second major "phase" of Medicare focused almost exclusively on controlling program costs. Indeed, soon after passage, many observers were already expressing concern at Medicare's growth. In 1970, then Chief Actuary Robert Myers predicted an enormous deficit in Medicare for 1995 (Myers 1970). Health care costs also received attention from President Richard Nixon during the period of wage and price controls. Predictions of Medicare's "bankruptcy" also began to surface. The 1981 report on the Federal Hospital Insurance Trust Fund indicated that the fund would be in deficit by 1991 (Board of Trustees 1981).

Worry over costs in the late 1970s spurred a number of cost-containment debates. However, the prospect of enormous federal deficits and efforts to reduce them provided the executive and legislative branches with additional impetus for major cost-containment measures in the following decade. By 1980, Medicare was the second largest federal domestic program and the fastest growing one, making it a target for those concerned about the size of government. Decisions about Medicare in the 1980s and 1990s reflected concern not only about rising health care costs but also about the size of the federal budget deficit.

Under each budget submission of the Reagan administration, Medicare cost cutting was accorded a central place in proposals to reduce the size of the federal budget deficit. Policy was as much budget-driven as centered on devising innovative approaches to provider payments. Nonetheless, many cost-containment strategies revolutionized the way we pay providers in the United States, and Medicare often has been used as a model for other payers seeking to hold down cost growth.

Enthusiasm for cost cutting within Medicare extended throughout the program. Most strategies emphasized reducing payments to Medicare service providers, but beneficiaries faced limitations on benefits and increased requirements for cost sharing. A study by the U.S. Congressional Budget Office (1991) concluded that, in 1990, Medicare spending was 20 percent below what it would have been without the changes of the 1980s. This helps to explain why the projected date of exhaustion of the Part A trust fund was extended in the 1980s (figure 2.4). Nonetheless, throughout the 1980s, Medicare was the fastest growing domestic federal program. In the 1990s, few cost-saving changes were passed until 1997, when major alterations in Medicare as part of the Balanced Budget Act helped balance the federal budget. As noted later in this chapter, nearly every part of Medicare faced changes under the BBA.

Hospital Reforms

From 1966 to 1974, Medicare paid hospitals on the principle of "reasonable and necessary costs." Hospitals had to fill out detailed cost reports and face auditing of their expenses, but they billed Medicare for whatever services they provided. These were not the published charges that hospitals generally apply to patients but were the costs for each hospital as calculated by Medicare's intermediaries—that is, private claims processors hired by Medicare. Hospitals could not charge whatever they liked, but once payment levels were established, there were no constraints on the amount of care provided.

Although this was the initial bargain struck to help Medicare pass, debate began almost immediately on how to control hospital costs. Robert Myers (1970) noted that even in the first several years of Medicare, there was interest in a per capita payment system for hospitals. But although the concern was there, consensus on major reform was lacking (Feder 1977).

A number of more limited constraints were introduced over this period. In 1972, professional standards review organizations (PSROs) were established to review and control beneficiaries' use of services (Feder et al. 1982). Beginning in 1974, a reimbursement cap was added to prevent any hospital from charging more than 120 percent of the mean of routine costs found in similar facilities. This first constraint on hospitals required them to hold costs in line with those of other nearby hospitals. Over time, this limit (called a "223" limit after its Social Security statute) was ratcheted downward to 112 percent (Office of Technology Assessment 1985). But this approach did not force major efficiencies on hospitals since they were still being paid on the basis of what they spent and the limits applied only to basic services.

In 1974 and 1975, Hospital Insurance payments grew at rates in excess of 20 percent, which prompted the Jimmy Carter administration to propose national hospital rate setting in the late 1970s (Feder et al. 1982). This dramatic proposal was defeated when hospitals pledged voluntarily to hold down costs. While considering rate-setting legislation, hospital cost growth slowed substantially, despite high inflation. But after the legislation failed, this "voluntary effort" had only temporarily reduced growth in hospital spending. In 1980 and 1981, growth rates in HI once more approached 20 percent, even though inflation was abating (figure 3.2). The industry could no longer credibly argue that it could police itself.

The confluence of efforts to cut Medicare spending as part of general budget reductions and concerns about rampant growth in the hospital sector made hospitals an obvious target for budget cuts. Since over two-thirds of Medicare payments went to hospitals, they were the place "where the money was." Medicare cost cutting for hospitals in the 1980s did not start with the prospective payment system (PPS), as many believe; its origins were earlier. The Omnibus Budget Reconciliation Act (OBRA) of 1981 tightened the 223 limits on what hospitals could receive as reimbursement for routine operating costs to 108 percent of mean costs (Office of Technology Assessment 1985). This first major effort to restrain costs in the 1980s focused on reducing payments to hospitals with high operating costs.

The Tax Equity and Fiscal Responsibility Act (TEFRA) of 1982 added substantially more stringent restrictions. TEFRA expanded the 223 lim-

Figure 3.2. Annual Rates of Growth in Medicare Hospital Payments, 1975–2004

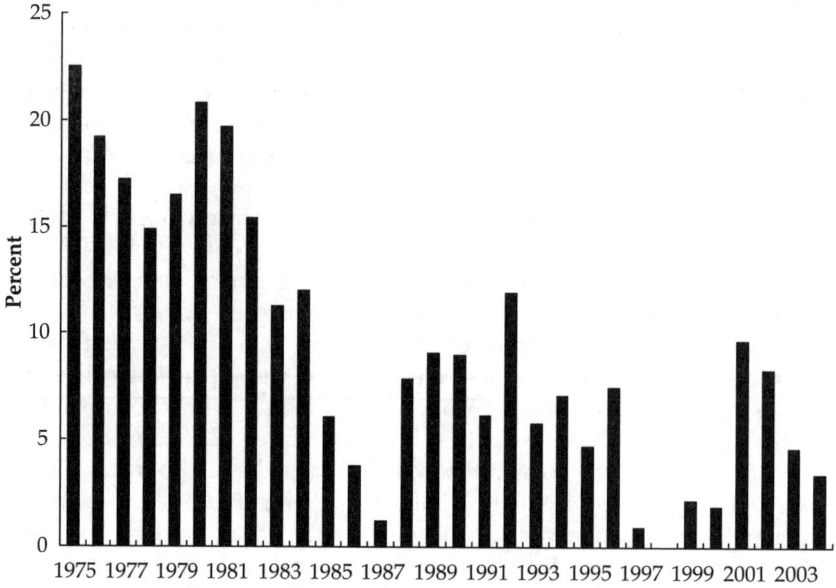

Sources: Board of Trustees, HI Trust Fund (1991, 1993, 1995, 2000, 2001, 2003, 2005).

its to cover more areas of spending. It also added a new hospital-specific target rate on growth in costs per case. But the most important change was that these limits would no longer be based on spending each year, but rather on costs up to a ceiling projected forward through time. This meant that each year the restrictions would be more severe and more binding (Office of Technology Assessment 1985). Consequently, impacts on spending growth were considerable (figure 3.2).

TEFRA also introduced several new concepts into hospital reimbursement. First, the payment growth limits moved away from payments based on what was spent on a particular patient to a payment schedule set in advance. TEFRA replaced the old per-diem approach to hospital payment with a per-case approach and permitted hospitals to benefit, at least partially, from any cost savings they generated. For the first time, hospitals had incentives to seek efficiencies in the provision of care, for example, by reducing lengths of stay per case. But the stringent TEFRA limits left hospitals without much flexibility to benefit from the efficiencies they introduced over time. The climate set by the TEFRA limits led many hospitals to conclude that almost any other plan would be preferable; this smoothed the way for introducing more radical payment reform.

The new hospital payment reform was implemented quickly. The U.S. Department of Health and Human Services (HHS) presented its proposal to Congress in December 1982, with many unresolved details left open for negotiation. Some pundits predicted that prolonged debate and lobbying would delay passage. But the Reagan administration and Congress worked feverishly in the spring of 1983 to hash out the compromise that led to the legislation. Although the HHS and the Congressional Budget Office put considerable effort into analyzing the impacts on hospitals of various alternatives, the deadlines for enactment dictated that many adjustments were ad hoc and many potential impacts remained unclear.

The new legislation, called the prospective payment system (PPS), came into being in April 1983. Because PPS was tied to critical legislation to protect the solvency of the Social Security system, the PPS amendments received less attention than if they had been proposed as standalone legislation. The final details were not debated or subjected to the scrutiny of interest groups, which might have slowed the process.

PPS began as a great experiment in systemwide reform, with no one certain of the outcome. In fact, Congress also established a prospective payment assessment commission (ProPAC) to oversee the implementation of this complicated new system and to advise on the inevitable changes necessary to finetune it over time.[13] PPS counts as a major coup for Congress and the administration. It radically changed payment policy to hospitals with a minimum of disruption to the health care system. Lengths of stay came down and care shifted to outpatient settings at a faster pace than would likely have happened without PPS.

After initial controversy, the system has become an accepted approach to establishing payments for hospitals. Rather than seeking to change the basic system, legislation has altered PPS by creating new hospital categories with specific adjustments to account for unusually high costs that the basic system cannot account for over time. Some of these adjustments address real inequities while others attempt to correct problems affecting hospitals that go well beyond the Medicare program. These adjustments have addressed the political needs of policymakers responding to complaints from rural hospitals, teaching hospitals, and hospitals that treat a disproportionate share of low-income patients. Further, raising payments each year based on a market basket of input costs has been a favorite tool for cost containment, ratcheting down the increase by a percentage point or two.

Physician Payment Reform

From the outset, the government encouraged physicians to participate in Medicare by setting generous initial payment levels and promising not to restrict the care doctors provide. For the first 20 years of Medicare, physician reimbursement went largely unchanged. But physician payment growth became a major issue in the 1980s, particularly as physician growth continued to spiral upward relative to hospital payments, which were moderating. Physicians also represented a target for cost-cutting efforts because of their high incomes and potential influence over health care spending.

Starting in 1984, payments were reduced through several mechanisms, including a freeze on how fast charges were allowed to grow. This fee freeze was instituted on July 1, 1984. The legislation permitted no increase in the "prevailing charge" for physicians—which served as the absolute upper bound on Medicare-allowed charges. Since this situation was analogous to the TEFRA changes that helped push PPS for hospitals, many felt that reform could be hammered out before the freeze was lifted. But consensus remained elusive, and Congress failed to enact broader reform. After one further extension, the freeze was finally lifted in May 1986. Despite the fee freeze, costs of the physician services' portion of Part B continued to grow rapidly. And physician payment reform took longer to accomplish.

Many policymakers had long expressed doubts about Medicare's Part B payment structure, arguing that it locked in historical inequities. These imbalances sent the wrong signals to physicians by paying more for expensive, high-technology services while offering few incentives for careful geriatric assessments or other basic care. Further, low payments in rural areas of the country discouraged physicians from practic-

Figure 3.3. Medicare Spending for Physician Services, 1993–2004

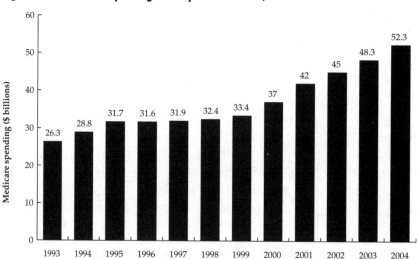

Sources: MedPAC (2004), Trustees Report (2005).

ing there. Finally, physician payments for the same services varied enormously around the country, and even within the same area—creating an extremely complex payment system that was not only difficult to manage but did not provide appropriate economic incentives to physicians. A new mechanism was needed. But any system that sought to change all these incentives would be controversial.

The desire to control costs and eliminate payment inequities led to debate about what approach to take. Some policymakers wanted the government to set fees and streamline the payment process; others sought more dramatic schemes to pay physicians, not on a fee-for-service basis but, rather, on a flat amount per patient (referred to as "capitation" approaches). Often, this latter approach focused on using formal groups such as health maintenance organizations (HMOs) to oversee the volume of all service use (not just physician services). The goal of simplifying the system so that it could be better controlled was also an important factor in the debate.

Fee reform may have stalled in the early 1980s, but recognition of the problem increased. In an attempt to speed reform consensus, Congress established a Physician Payment Review Commission (PPRC) in 1986 and charged it with hammering out the details of a reform package to propose to Congress and the Reagan administration. In March 1987, the PPRC recommended a resource-based relative value scale (RBRVS) approach (PPRC 1987). That is, each service was given its own index value that would reflect differences in the resources necessary to provide the services; then, each year, a base fee ("conversion factor") would be established to translate the index numbers into specific fees. The PPRC noted that this would not rule out further moves away from a fee-based system; rather, the fee schedule was emphasized as a necessary first step. Some in the Reagan administration remained skeptical of relying only on a fee schedule and preferred more radical change to move away from a fee-for-service approach. Nonetheless, the Health Care Financing Administration (HCFA), now known as the Centers for Medicare and Medicaid Services, funded a major study of the RBRVS approach (Hsiao et al. 1988) that laid the groundwork for creating the value of each service relative to a base.

Debate continued until 1989, when Congress, at the eleventh hour, passed the Medicare fee schedule as part of the Omnibus Budget Reconciliation Act of 1989, using the RBRVS approach. Like the PPS, this change was combined with other more comprehensive legislation. A gradual transition to this new payment system began on January 1, 1992. The fee schedule did not reduce the overall level of payments to physicians (i.e., it was promised to be "budget neutral"), but it did reduce payments for surgeries and procedures (which were deemed "overvalued") while increasing payments for basic office visits.

Implementation of the fee schedule was not smooth, however. Doctors expressed outrage at a preemptive strike on reform through a 1990 budget agreement that essentially instituted some of the cuts in the "overvalued" procedures without offsetting increases in "undervalued" ones. But they exploded over an even more controversial issue that arose with the release of proposed regulations for the fee schedule in the summer of 1991. The initial starting value (the "conversion factor") for the fee schedule was to be adjusted downward resulting in a 16.5 percent cut from what it otherwise would have been. The reason for the adjustment was the prediction that doctors would increase the volume of their services and so the fees needed to be set lower to offset potential new spending. Doctors, led by the AMA, argued that volume adjustments should not be made and that they would adversely affect payment levels. For example, HCFA calculated that an intermediate office visit for an established patient would rise only from $26 in 1991 before the fee schedule to $27 in 1992—not much of an increase for a fee that the schedule presumably sought to favor. There would be little good news in fees to offset the bad news for specialists. The promise of "budget neutrality" meant different things to the government and to doctors. The government wanted to ensure that total reimbursements to physicians would not rise, while physicians' representatives were looking at the issue on a fee-by-fee basis.

After much acrimony and threatened congressional intervention, HCFA produced its final regulations in November of 1991. The agency softened the cut in the conversion factor. As a consequence, that same intermediate office visit would now rise to $30 in 1992, rather than $27. This also softened the blow for procedures scheduled to be cut. For example, coronary artery bypass surgery would have fallen from $3,178 in 1991 to $2,726 in 1992 under the June rules, but only to $2,892 under the November rules.

In retrospect, the physicians' concerns proved correct since rates of growth in spending were lower than projected. No large increase in volume—as the government had feared—happened. Just as was the case with PPS, physicians did not immediately act to "game" the system by increasing the volume of visits. In fact, spending growth slowed (figure 3.3). Over time, other payers have adopted the idea of the RBRVS.

Since 1992, a number of further changes have been applied to the fee schedule, and it has become less true to its original goals compared with the PPS. Many of the new codes added to the system have been for procedures by specialists, and these codes tend to carry higher values. As a consequence, the relative differences between primary and specialty care have declined.

The way annual payment increases are established has also changed over time. Early attempts tying payment increases to the general volume of services were jettisoned. The current update formula is called the sustainable growth rate system (SGR) and ties updates to several factors, including growth in the national economy. Another factor is aggregate physician volume, which is influenced by use per beneficiary and the number of beneficiaries in the fee-for-service portion of the program. While the economy grew rapidly in the late 1990s and early 2000s, payment levels rose faster than inflation (MedPAC 2003). But when the economic downturn occurred and beneficiaries dropped out of HMOs and returned to fee-for-service Medicare, the SGR formula called for declines in payment levels. Remedial legislation has largely overturned those declines, but changes in the SGR to alter the update formula permanently have not yet occurred. This area of physician payment remains controversial and likely will continue to be examined yearly since projections indicate that fees will continue to decline unless further adjustments are made.

Other Budget Reduction Efforts before 1997

Although most of the cost-containment attention has been directed at inpatient hospital and physician services, which represent the biggest shares of Medicare, other areas have also been subject to budget reductions. Indeed, the effort has been so extensive that micromanagement of budget cutting reached new heights in the 1990 budget deal. To achieve $43 billion in five-year savings, almost no part of Medicare remained unscathed. For example, laboratory fees were reduced, payments for prosthetic devices were frozen, and further restrictions were added to the coverage of seat-lift chairs and power scooters. These changes produced only a tiny portion of the $43 billion savings but spread the pain across many providers.

During the 1980s, additional areas were subject to substantial cost-saving efforts. For example, home health care and skilled nursing facility (SNF) benefits initially were constrained by regulations and later by new payment systems. Home health and SNF benefits have always been limited to skilled-care needs to keep them from becoming benefits for general long-term care services.

The first of these two service areas, home health, has gone through numerous expansions and contractions. Home health services are a medical benefit available to enrollees under the care of a physician, confined to home, and needing skilled nursing services on an intermittent basis. Coverage is also available for those who need physical or speech therapy (and have met other criteria). The coinsurance requirement for home health was removed in 1972, and further liberalization in 1980 eliminated the deductible, a 100-day limit, and a prior hospitalization requirement. In addition, in 1980, proprietary agencies were permitted to operate without licensing requirements, leading to a rapid expansion in the supply of home health services—which likely had the greatest impact on use of services (Kenney 1991).

When reimbursement for home health services grew more than 25 percent a year from 1980 to 1983, HCFA scrutinized intermediaries' adherence to the eligibility requirements and types of services received. HCFA clamped down on activities and instructed intermediaries to examine claims closely. Denial rates increased (Leader and Moon 1989) and the rate of growth of reimbursements slowed—even though the introduction of PPS was expected to cause hospitals to discharge patients earlier and thus accelerate the use of home health services. In 1984, HCFA issued new guidelines to fiscal intermediaries regarding part-time and intermittent requirements. The 1984 guidelines required that an otherwise eligible individual would qualify for the benefit only if the care were both part-time (less than eight hours per day) *and* intermittent (four or fewer days per week). Eligibility also required that the individual be homebound. This was a catch-22; the individual had to be incapacitated but well enough to need only part-time care. The regulatory strategy to hold down costs proved effective. By 1988, the rate of growth in reimbursements slowed to 1.1 percent and declined in 1987 (U.S. Congress, Committee on Ways and Means 1991).

Then in 1989, an important lawsuit, *Duggan v. Bowen*, eased these requirements substantially. The definitions of medical necessity changed, the definition of intermittency was relaxed, and the guidelines to intermediaries were rewritten to establish consistent treatment. The result was an enormous expansion of services beginning in 1989 and lasting until after the 1997 changes described below (see figure 3.4). Between 1989 and 1994, Medicare spending on home health increased fivefold and, by 1994, accounted for 8 percent of all Medicare spending. Rates of growth over this period averaged almost 37 percent annually— a rate of growth more than three times that of the rest of the Medicare program. Most of this expansion occurred from greater use of services rather than higher payment levels. Between 1988 and 1994, the proportion of beneficiaries receiving home health services nearly doubled and the average number of visits per user almost tripled (Kenney and Moon 1995). Much of the growth in visits occurred for persons receiving 100 or more visits, shifting this service more toward a long-term care benefit. As discussed below, the growth in the 1990s made home health a target for further change in 1997.

Like home health care, skilled nursing facility (SNF) care has always been constrained by its definition. SNF benefits are restricted to enrollees who have had a three-day prior hospital stay and who need skilled nursing or rehabilitation services. In 1969, SNF benefits were limited to enrollees on a course of recovery. These limitations restricted the

Figure 3.4. Medicare Spending for Post-Acute Care, by Setting, 1992–2003

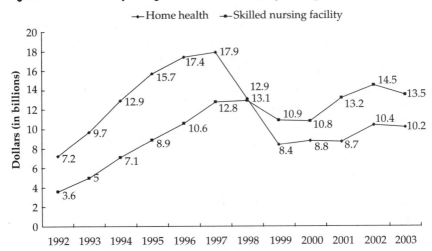

Sources: MedPAC (2004); CMS, Office of the Actuary (2003).

persons eligible and ensured that Medicare never became a substantial provider of long-term care (Smits, Feder, and Scanlon 1982). In addition, until the late 1980s, intermediaries had regulatory discretion over duration of benefits and what conditions qualified people for SNF reimbursement; these interpretations varied widely across the United States (Liu and Kenney 1991). Earlier studies criticized the arbitrary and after-the-fact rulings about coverage that discouraged nursing home participation (Smits et al. 1982). Nonetheless, these rulings operated as an important cost constraint on SNF care and became more important during the mid-1980s when PPS encouraged earlier hospital discharges. Perhaps the most crucial cost-control force, however, was the relatively low reimbursement rates under Medicare.

In the 1980s, cost-sharing requirements became more severe. Up to 100 days of SNF services are covered by Medicare, but cost sharing is assessed against days 21 through 100. Moreover, the level of the required co-payment is tied to the hospital deductible, which rose rapidly in the 1980s and outpaced the growth in the costs of SNF care. In fact, at one-eighth of the hospital deductible, SNF cost sharing turned out to be nearly as high as the daily payment to some providers of SNF care at the end of the 1980s. Consequently, for many beneficiaries, the SNF benefit essentially became only a 20-day benefit (Liu and Kenney 1991), with other private arrangements made after that. This was yet another force keeping growth down without formal policy change.

The situation changed substantially in 1988 when a legal ruling established more uniform coverage guidelines, removing a barrier to receiving care. Much of the discretion intermediaries employed in interpreting what services were covered was eliminated. Consequently, heavy-care patients, such as those requiring tube feeding, became eligible for the first time (Liu and Kenney 1991). SNF reimbursements jumped upward, a movement that continued in 1989 with the addition of benefits from the Medicare Catastrophic Coverage Act (described in chapter 4). The SNF expansions from that legislation were later repealed, but SNF use did not return to its earlier levels of low growth due in part to the large numbers of nursing facilities that geared up to serve Medicare patients in 1989. Expenditures grew from $2.5 billion in 1990 to $9.0 billion in 1995, more than tripling in five years.

Savings in other areas have been a bit more elusive. Outpatient hospital services, which have grown enormously since the program began, received considerable attention and some cost cutting, but major policy change did not occur in this area until 1997. Payment policy for outpatient services remained a hodgepodge of ad hoc adjustments (Sulvetta 1992), with scheduled payment reform delayed several times. Congress first mandated recommendations from HCFA in 1989 (U.S. Congress, Committee on Ways and Means 1989). In 1997, prospective payment systems were added for outpatient hospital care, home health services, and SNF services. Even then, it took years before the new systems came online.

HEALTH MAINTENANCE ORGANIZATIONS

Since 1983, Medicare has allowed health maintenance organizations (HMOs) to contract with the government to serve beneficiaries in exchange for a set monthly payment. HMOs then take on the risk of providing the full range of Medicare benefits to those who enroll. This option, designed to allow Medicare to take advantage of managed care, promised to control costs by overseeing the full range of services delivered. It also made the costs to Medicare more predictable because HMOs are paid a fixed amount per beneficiary per month regardless of use of services.

Enrollment in HMOs initially grew rapidly, albeit from a very small base. In 1985, only 3.6 percent of Medicare beneficiaries were enrolled in some type of HMO (Health Care Financing Administration [HCFA] 1995). By 1987, enrollment grew by more than 50 percent. After that it leveled off and reached only 2 million by 1991. Since that time, the number of beneficiaries signing up for HMOs has increased dramatically. By the end of 1995, 3.8 million were enrolled. However, enrollment remained spotty; large shares of enrollees signed up in Southern California, Florida, Oregon, and New York, while vast parts of the country had little or no Medicare HMO penetration. Medicare HMO enrollment also continued to lag behind the move toward managed care for the nonelderly population.

A period of rapid growth began again after 1995. In 1999, enrollment in these private plans reached a peak of 6.2 million beneficiaries or about 16 percent of the Medicare population (Boards of Trustees 2005). Noting this rapid growth, many observers became concerned that payments to private plans were set so high that the plans were able to offer substantially more services than what was available in traditional Medicare.

As a result, there was considerable controversy over whether the HMO program was generating any savings for Medicare. The essential step in generating savings is determining how to pay HMOs—a critical factor in ensuring that competition among plans occurs fairly. Originally, Medicare based its payment on an estimate of the average amount it would have spent on beneficiaries if they had remained in the traditional fee-for-service program. The amount (referred to as the adjusted average per capita cost, or AAPCC) was calculated for each county in the United States and reflected differences by age, gender, and whether the beneficiary was institutionalized. Medicare then paid 95 percent of that amount to generate savings for the program. But savings could only result if the AAPCC was less than what those enrolling would otherwise have cost Medicare.

Studies of Medicare HMOs concluded that healthier-than-average beneficiaries—or at least those who used less than an average amount of health services—were more likely to enroll. HMOs attracted Medicare beneficiaries selectively, enrolling beneficiaries whose average costs were lower than Medicare's per capita payment because they were low-risk patients. As a result, the HMO program was more expensive for the government than if those beneficiaries had remained in traditional Medicare (Langwell and Hadley 1989). The most comprehensive study found that Medicare beneficiaries enrolled in HMOs only cost about 89 percent of the average (Brown et al. 1993). This meant that each new enrollee in an HMO, on average, increased, not decreased, costs to the program. Later studies have also found that HMO enrollment increases costs to the government.

THE BALANCED BUDGET ACT OF 1997

The Balanced Budget Act of 1997 (BBA) eclipsed all earlier efforts at holding down costs in Medicare. Although Medicare changes constituted only part of the legislation, Medicare's cuts were disproportionately large, and it is not an exaggeration to say that the federal budget would not have been balanced had it not been for the changes in Medicare. Moreover, once the changes were put in place, they proved to have an even larger impact than anticipated, leading to some later softening of the changes that were made.

The initial projections were for $116.4 billion in net spending reductions over the five years after enactment.[14] Over ten years, savings were expected to total $393.8 billion. Overall, annual per capita rate of growth on spending under the Medicare program was projected to go from the 6.5 percent anticipated over 10 years to less than 5.3 percent annually. The BBA was expected to extend the life of the Part A trust fund, delaying the date of exhaustion from 2001 to 2007—another important accomplishment. Further, the BBA led the Board of Trustees to substantially lower projections of Medicare as a share of gross domestic product (GDP) between 1997 and 1998 (figure 3.5). The combined share of Part A and Part B spending went from a 1997 projection of 6.5 percent of GDP in 2025 to a projected level of 5.3 percent in the 1998 report (Board of Trustees 1997, 1998).

In the first five years, the largest share of Medicare savings were to come from reductions in payments to hospitals. But over 10 years, hospital changes were expected to be smaller than savings from the private plan payment reductions, and about the same size as the increase in Part B premiums. Altogether, reductions in payments under the traditional fee-for-service portion of the program were expected to

Figure 3.5. Projected 2025 Medicare Spending as a Share of GDP

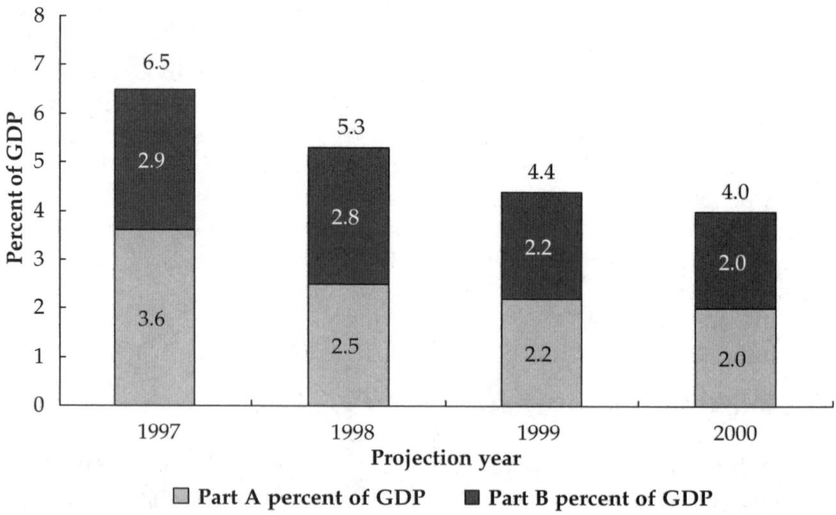

■ Part A percent of GDP   ■ Part B percent of GDP

Source: Board of Trustees (1997–2000).

account for over two-thirds of the savings in the first five years and over half of the savings over the 10-year period. From the perspective of the Medicare program and its beneficiaries, some changes were improvements in policy, but others generated problems.

In practice, determining the exact amount of savings is difficult (since factors such as changes in the health care system and the numbers of persons drawing benefits do not remain constant over time). Also during this period, efforts to curb Medicare fraud and abuse increased, growth in overall health care spending slowed, and GDP grew faster than expected. Each of these likely helped slow program growth. Nonetheless, the BBA's impact was certainly much greater than anticipated— the average rate of growth in Medicare from 1997 to 2003 slowed to an annual rate of 4.6 percent, compared with the 1997 projections of 6.5 percent—a 41 percent reduction.

Another way to examine how the actual impact of the BBA varied compared with projections done right after its passage is to measure the projected share of GDP that Medicare would require in the future. In the Trustees reports for 1999 and 2000, projected shares of GDP continued to decline as a result of greater-than-expected impacts from the BBA. In the 1999 projections, the share was expected to be 2.3 percent for 2025, compared with 6.5 percent projected in 1997. In the 2000 Trustees report, the projected GDP share again changed, but just to 4 percent of GDP. This was still substantially lower than the 1997 figure. Some of this increase reflects changes made by Congress to moderate the BBA's effects on Medicare providers in 1998 and 1999 (Board of Trustees 2000).

This downward trend in projected shares of GDP improved substantially the outlook for Medicare. Indeed, the date of exhaustion of the Part A trust fund was extended from 2001 in the 1997 projections to 2025 in the 2000 projections (Board of Trustees 2000). Again, the Part A trust fund outlook reflected not only lower projected expenditures but higher expected payroll taxes from an economy that performed beyond expectations.

Changes to the Traditional Program

A majority of the Medicare savings in the Balanced Budget Act came from reductions in provider payments in the traditional fee-for-service program, mainly by limiting the growth rates for hospital payments. Although the fee-for-service changes were quite large, most of them were not controversial, at least initially. Restructuring the payment methods for rehabilitation hospitals, home health agencies, skilled nursing facilities, and outpatient services provided a second major source of savings. Physician services were treated rather lightly.

Hospital payments accounted for about 44 percent of all Medicare expenditures in 1997 and represented almost 30 percent of the expected savings over five years. Half of the savings from hospitals were from reductions in the update factors for hospitals under PPS. In addition to the across-the-board changes, teaching facilities and hospitals serving a disproportionate share of low-income Medicare beneficiaries were subject to additional limits in payment growth. PPS-exempt hospitals, such as rehabilitation facilities; long-term care hospitals; psychiatric, children's, and cancer hospitals; and hospice facilities also had their update factors that determined annual rates of increase reduced.

New payment systems also changed the traditional program for home health, skilled nursing care, and outpatient services. The move away from a cost-based system improved incentives for service providers to reduce costs. Further, payments moved away from per-service levels. For example, home health payments were shifted to an episode-of-care basis (after an interim policy reduced the use of services). The net result was a decline in spending on home health services in 1998 and 1999, and modest expansions since then (figure 3.4). In 2003, spending on home health services was $10.2 billion and about $12 billion in 2005, still below the maximum reached in 1996 of $16.8 billion.

While skilled nursing care continued to be reimbursed on a per-diem basis, payments were consolidated across services to give a predetermined rate for each day of care, adjusted by the health status of the patient (referred to as a "case mix adjustment"). Patients were assigned to 44 groups depending upon service needs and likelihood of resource use. Adopted in 1998, the PPS still adjusts payment levels for local market conditions. The PPS has had problems, however, largely due to questions about the groupings, particularly for patients with extensive needs. Later legislation increased payment levels for various groups. Spending on SNF care has also been lower than expected since the BBA.

Outpatient service payments were also changed, creating a PPS that went into effect in August 2000. The outpatient PPS operates on a calendar year basis and initially updates were linked to the hospital market basket. Like the physician PPS, the outpatient hospital system sets payment rates for individual services on a set of relative weights, a conversion factor, and an adjustment for geographic differences in input prices. The various procedures are classified into 570 ambulatory payment classifications (APCs). Items that are clinically similar and use comparable amounts of services are grouped together (MedPAC 2003b).

In total, the BBA gained a substantial portion of its savings from reduced growth in the fee-for-service program. Although some opportunities to further improve the program were lost in conference, overall, these changes improved Medicare's payment policies. Critics, however, argued that reductions in areas like home health services went too far, and adjustments relaxing the reductions have been made since 1997.

Private Plan Changes

Private plan changes included reductions in the growth of payment levels and the creation of a new set of options. As the conference language made clear, Congress believed it set in motion "the first defined contribution plan in which beneficiaries may enroll,"[15] signaling the significance conferees attached to these changes. In addition, requirements designed to improve beneficiary information and modify geographic adjustments to the payment structure were also important elements of the BBA. Even the name of this option changed to Medicare-+Choice.

Savings from this part of the Medicare program were expected to total $22.5 billion over five years and $97 billion over 10 years from a slowdown in payments made to private plans. They reflected a combination of the indirect effects of savings in the traditional fee-for-service side of the program—since those costs served as the basis for establishing private plan payments—and of a further reduction in the annual update of payments to private plans over and above the fee-for-service-driven changes.[16]

The Balanced Budget Act introduced several new types of plans from which Medicare beneficiaries could choose. The most controversial new type was the medical savings account (MSA) where beneficiaries would be able to enroll in a high deductible plan, with any positive difference between the Medicare contribution and the cost of the policy deposited in a medical savings account. Provider-sponsored organizations were less controversial in terms of their offerings and consumer protections, but are also estimated to result in higher costs to the Medicare program as a result of favorable risk selection. A third addition to the private plan options was unrestricted fee-for-service plans. The overall concern expressed at passage—especially for the MSA option—was whether these plans would create risk selection problems, attracting healthier individuals. In practice, there has been very little private sector interest in offering these MSA plans.

The most important part of this legislation turned out to be the lowered annual updates in payment levels that effectively limited payment increases to 2 percent per year. This new payment system was also intended to move away from any direct link to fee-for-service spending levels and provide an improved risk adjustment mechanism.

A last major element in the BBA affecting private plans was an effort to reduce the large variations in payments to plans in different parts of the country. In areas where the payments were very low—as low as $221 per month in 1997—private plans simply had not developed. So one goal of the legislation was to reduce these differences to enhance the development of managed care options in rural areas. New payment floors were established, guaranteeing higher payments in low-cost areas.

Although the intent of these changes was clearly to stimulate growth in the number of private plans, the opposite occurred. Very few new types of plans ever emerged and the rural floors did little to attract new plans. On the other hand, the slower growth in payments to plans over time took a major toll. Enrollment declined as plans withdrew from participation and others cut back on services. Heavy lobbying by the industry restored some payments in the early 2000s, and the drug legislation once again upped payments substantially (see chapter 4). But enrollment has not returned to the levels achieved before the BBA led to major withdrawals.

Changes in Beneficiary Contributions

The only major change in required beneficiary contributions the BBA made was to increase the Part B premium. Two changes were put in place: the first permanently set the Part B premium at 25 percent of the costs of Part B services to elderly beneficiaries. The second change shifted almost all home health services from Part A to Part B, thereby raising Part B spending and increasing the premiums required of beneficiaries. These two changes affecting Part B premiums were a significant part of the overall benefit reduction package, expected to achieve 13 percent of all Medicare savings over five years and 24 percent over 10 years.

Protections for low-income beneficiaries from the substantially higher Part B premiums were included in the BBA through an extension of the programs run by Medicaid to protect low-income individuals from high cost sharing and premiums. The new Qualified Individuals program was a capped entitlement, meaning that not all beneficiaries eligible were guaranteed protection. Persons with incomes between 120 and 175 percent of the federal poverty level *might* receive protections ranging from the full cost of the Part B premium to protections only against the home health premium increase. Like other low-income protections, the number of persons receiving these benefits remained limited. (The benefit for individuals with income from 135 to 175 percent of the poverty level lapsed in 2002.)

Other changes also affected beneficiaries. Expansions in preventive services—such as more frequent mammography, diabetes management services, and bone density and colorectal cancer screening—expanded

Medicare's benefit package and help offset higher required contributions. In addition, beneficiaries using hospital outpatient services were helped by a gradual reduction in co-payments to the 20 percent commonly associated with other Part B services. Other changes, however, increased beneficiary costs. In particular, the savings planned for private plan options came in part from higher premiums and fewer extra benefits available to those enrolling in the private options.

4

HOW MEDICARE HAS CHANGED: BENEFITS

The basic benefit structure for Medicare has been changed only incrementally since the program began, with two exceptions: the Medicare Catastrophic Coverage Act of 1988 (MCCA), which was repealed just over a year after its initial passage, and the Medicare Prescription Drug, Improvement, and Modernization Act of 2003 (MMA), which is currently being implemented. These two pieces of legislation created substantial expansions in Medicare benefits. Other changes have been very modest and usually have affected the level of cost sharing or premiums that beneficiaries must pay. This chapter first notes the modest changes over time and then turns to the contrasts in legislative strategies presented by MCCA and MMA.

INCREMENTAL CHANGES IN MEDICARE BENEFITS

Before the 2003 legislation created a drug benefit, the only new types of benefits Medicare covered were the hospice benefit and a modest set of preventive services added at several times over the years.[1]

The Medicare hospice benefit was started in 1983 for persons whose doctor certifies that, if their illness runs its normal course, are expected to die within six months. The benefit covers a broad set of palliative services including skilled nursing and homemaker services, therapy, physicians' services, counseling, and medical social services. Care is usually delivered in the patient's home but may also include hospital and institutional care. Prescription drugs for the treatment of pain are covered under hospice at a modest co-pay of 5 percent. This benefit began on a very small scale, and although enrollment has increased considerably in the 2000s, it is still quite limited. For example, spending on hospice grew from $3.5 billion in 2001 to $5.9 billion in 2003, a 30 percent annual increase (MedPAC 2004a). In 2003, the hospice benefit served a little more than half a million beneficiaries.

Preventive services have also been gradually added to Medicare over time. In general, the list is limited to services for which there is medical evidence of effectiveness and a prescribed frequency of use. A partial list includes mammograms, pap smears, colonoscopies, diabetes eye exams, glaucoma screenings, and flu and pneumonia immunizations. In addition to covering these services, Medicare sometimes waives the deductible and co-pay amounts.

Benefits have also changed in the treatment of premiums and cost sharing. As chapter 1 indicated, Medicare has a complicated cost-sharing structure with big differences between Parts A and B. For example, since 1966, the Part A deductible has risen from $40 to $952 in 2006 because it is tied to the costs of hospital care. Since an annual adjustment was established by law, this increase does not reflect a legislative change. Part B's deductible, on the other hand, was initially set higher than Part A at $50. But it was increased only a few times and its level was not linked to any index until 2005. In 2006, it is $124. (The new drug legislation established an index for the deductible, so it will continue to rise in the future.) Cost-sharing rules have changed for the home health program when cost sharing was eliminated in 1972. Other changes have also been made over time (mainly in 1972) that expanded access to home health care.

Premiums for Part B have also undergone important changes. Originally the premium was set at 50 percent of the costs of Part B services. But health care spending—particularly under Part B—grew so much more rapidly than Social Security benefits that the premiums began taking up more and more of the monthly Social Security benefit. As a consequence, in 1972, the premium was tied to the rate of growth of Social Security benefits. Under these rules, in only eight years, the premium's share of Part B Medicare costs fell to 25 percent. Since lawmakers sought savings in the Medicare program, ad hoc changes to keep the premium at 25 percent of Part B services were passed, each lasting several years. The Balanced Budget Act of 1997 formally set the amount at 25 percent. Interestingly, although the premium was technically cut in half, its level compared with all of Medicare (Parts A and B) declined by much less—from 15.5 percent in 1970 to 9.4

percent in 2003 (Boards of Trustees 2004). This occurred because of the growth of Part B services relative to Part A over time. The Part B premium will continue to rise as a share of Medicare as Part B services grow more rapidly.

THE MEDICARE CATASTROPHIC COVERAGE ACT

The Medicare Catastrophic Coverage Act (MCCA) was one of the shortest-lived pieces of social legislation in the United States. It also marked a turning point in Medicare policy. Unlike earlier additions, such as the 1972 amendments that added new categories of eligible people, lowered the Part B premium, and expanded home health care benefits, the MCCA was intended to be budget neutral to the federal government, requiring beneficiaries to fund the additional benefits from higher premiums. Of particular note, part of the financing included an income-related premium. It also constituted a marked departure from earlier legislation proposed by the Reagan administration that sought to restrict Medicare coverage and reduce costs at the expense of both providers and beneficiaries. The MCCA sought to expand Medicare benefits, but in the context of the constraints faced by any legislation in the 1980s that defied the high federal deficit and the Gramm-Rudman-Hollings budget restrictions to expand the role of government. As such, it must be viewed in a broader political context as well.

The MCCA offers important political and economic lessons. In political terms, the act launched an unprecedented debate about the future of Medicare—one that continues today. Economically, it became clear that even minor changes in Medicare come with large price tags and that beneficiaries may not find the cost worth the perceived benefits when asked to pay for new benefits.

By 1987, cost sharing had increased to the point where elderly beneficiaries were spending nearly the same share of their incomes on health care as they did before Medicare was introduced (see chapter 1, figure 1.3). A considerable portion of that burden came from the rising deductible and coinsurance requirements of Medicare, as well as increasing costs for critical services that Medicare did not cover. When the MCCA was first debated, persons age 65 and over had average per capita expenditures of $5,360 on health care, only $3,356 of which came from public sources (i.e., Medicare and Medicaid) (Waldo et al. 1989), implying average out-of-pocket or premium expenses of just over $2,000. For example, the elderly were liable for nearly a quarter of the costs of hospital and physician services ($726 in 1987), which are relatively well covered by Medicare. The elderly also lacked coverage for nursing home care—their largest source of uncovered services—and for other crucial health care expenditures such as prescription drugs, dental care, and vision care.

These averages do not capture how high the liabilities can be for persons with even modest health problems. For example, individuals who trigger hospital coinsurance (meaning they had substantial stays) had an average out-of-pocket spending for Medicare-covered cost sharing of $7,852 in 1988 (U.S. Congressional Budget Office [CBO] 1987). Beneficiaries who did not trigger the coinsurance but had at least two hospital stays averaged $2,387 in Medicare cost-sharing liabilities, not counting spending on other health care services that Medicare does not cover. Many observers felt it was time to expand Medicare coverage to limit such high liabilities.

Setting the Stage for the Legislation

The Medicare Catastrophic Coverage Act owed its initial political impetus to the Bowen Commission—a group headed by former Secretary of Health and Human Services Otis Bowen. President Reagan had charged the Commission with studying problems associated with catastrophic health expenses, including both acute and long-term care for persons of all ages. The Bowen report, released in the fall of 1986, only proposed legislation to deal with the problem of gaps in acute care for Medicare beneficiaries (U.S. Department of Health and Human Services 1986). This issue was viewed as the "easiest" to solve of the major health care access problems because it was likely to be the least expensive and require only marginal changes. The original Bowen proposal called for a simple expansion of benefits financed with a flat $59 annual premium assessed on all Medicare enrollees. This was to be added to the existing Part B premium, fully covering the costs of the program. The benefit improvement would consist of an annual $2,000 limit on each beneficiary's out-of-pocket expenses arising from hospital and physician deductibles and coinsurance. Once the beneficiary paid $2,000, the Medicare program would forgive all further Medicare cost sharing under both Parts A and B in that calendar year, regardless of beneficiary income and assets. In addition, hospital cost sharing would be limited to no more than two deductibles per year. Otherwise, Medicare would remain the same. This simple proposal added so-called "stop-loss" protection to Medicare similar to that found in many employer-covered policies.

The willingness of the Reagan administration to support a $2 billion expansion in Medicare benefits took many by surprise. But with White House support came a number of stringent constraints—namely, that new benefits must be self-financed by the beneficiaries and that the financing must come from beneficiary premiums rather than from general taxes. The proposed flat premium of about $5 per month was to be a straightforward increase in insurance coverage. Although the bill would expand the scope of government benefits, it would not expand subsidies to elderly and disabled persons. Capitol Hill staffers and interest groups such as the AARP began to develop their own versions of the legislation, but worked within the requirement of having beneficiaries bear the full costs. Even within this framework, the contents of the benefit package were soon transformed. The Democrats in Congress took on a tough challenge: enhance the benefits while adhering to the constraint of self-financing through premiums. How much could be added without risking a presidential veto?

Defining the Benefits and Financing

During the spring of 1987, a number of modest additions to Bowen's package began to surface. For example, an early draft from the House Committee on Ways and Means added a limit on Part B out-of-pocket liabilities and simplified the hospital benefit. Proposed changes in home health and skilled nursing facility (SNF) care were viewed as minor improvements in long-term care.

Later, the House of Representatives made two other broad additions. First, major Medicaid expansions were added to provide relief from Medicare coinsurance and deductibles for the low-income elderly, as well as to improve financial protection for spouses of nursing home residents.[2] The first of these changes required that Medicaid pay coinsurance, deductibles, and premiums for all Medicare-covered services for beneficiaries with incomes below the federal poverty level. This added further protections for low-income beneficiaries without differentiating coverage within the Medicare program itself. It also protected the lowest-income beneficiaries from the new higher premiums. The second change relaxed income and asset limits on spouses of persons in nursing homes, making more people eligible for Medicaid benefits.

Other provisions in the legislation effectively freed up the funds to pay for these Medicaid provisions. That is, when Medicare's coverage became more generous with limits on total cost sharing ("stop-loss") and other protections, Medicaid costs for persons already covered by both programs would fall and states' burdens for the over-65 and disabled populations would be eased, allowing states to provide the new Medicaid benefits without requiring new state revenues. By expanding Medicaid in this way, the MCCA sought to prevent states from reducing their own health care spending in response to the new provisions.

The second major expansion added drug coverage to the package. In part, this was viewed as a way to offer benefits to higher-income enrollees who were being asked to pay a disproportionate share of the costs of the legislation (discussed below). This change established an entirely new benefit. But to keep it a "catastrophic" benefit (i.e., restricted to those with well above average health care expenses), there would be a high deductible before Medicare would begin to pay. Even so, a substantial number of Medicare beneficiaries would qualify. Many advocates of this drug coverage expected older persons to view it as a major improvement in Medicare.

The Senate Finance Committee proceeded more cautiously than the House, but within a very similar framework. Its final package looked like a scaled-down version of the House bill but without the drug benefit. A July 1987 CBO study estimated the average annual benefits per enrollee at $78 for Bowen's version and $226 for the House version.

These benefit escalations created a major problem on the financing side. Although $5 per month might not be viewed as unduly burdensome on those with modest incomes, a $20 increase added to the already escalating Part B premium from the House version could hurt those it presumably sought to help: the modest-income elderly who would have trouble paying this new premium. Some other means of financing the benefit became imperative. Consequently, both the House and Senate proposed a smaller flat premium increase for everyone plus an income-related premium for those with incomes above a certain level. The term *supplemental premium* was carefully chosen to distinguish it from a tax increase. It was to be administered through the Internal Revenue Service (IRS), however, and paid using the 1040 form, making it seem to taxpayers suspiciously like a tax.

Passage

The Medicare Catastrophic Coverage Act passed in June of 1988 was hailed as "the largest expansion of Medicare since the program's establishment in 1965" (Torres-Gil 1989). A major ceremony was held in the Rose Garden of the White House on July 1, 1988, to celebrate its signing by President Ronald Reagan. In private, the drafters' enthusiasm was considerably lower—reflecting the long road of compromises necessary to enact such legislation.

On the Part A side, the legislation reduced beneficiaries' liability for hospital care to only one deductible per year and eliminated hospital coinsurance. Hospital benefits would now cover the full year.[3] This expansion and simplification of hospital coverage represented one of the more valuable benefit changes of the act; these benefits became effective in January 1989.

Also on the Part A side, the SNF benefit was made more generous by eliminating the requirement of a three-day prior hospital stay, lengthening the coverage to 150 days per year, and reducing and rearranging the coinsurance charged. Coinsurance would be required for the first eight days—but at a much lower rate of 20 percent of the daily cost of nursing home care (compared with a higher rate starting on day 21). These changes meant more beneficiaries would qualify for coverage and longer stays would be covered. Relaxing requirements on participation in these areas also modestly expanded hospice and home health benefits.

On the Part B side, the major expansion was intended to limit the amount of deductibles and co-payments beneficiaries would pay for physician and other services, for the first time placing a cap on how much Medicare beneficiaries pay out of pocket for Part B coinsurance and deductibles. Above the cap, Medicare would have paid the full 100 percent of allowed charges. This cap was scheduled to start at $1,370 in 1990 and, had the legislation not been repealed, would have risen each year at a rate intended to protect the 7 percent of enrollees with the highest Part B costs. The main beneficiaries of this stop-loss would have been persons undergoing surgeries or other very expensive medical procedures.

The major new addition to Medicare services was to be the drug benefit, covering outpatient prescription drugs above a $600 deductible. This very large deductible was also designed to limit the benefit to users with unusually high liabilities. It was scheduled to rise each year to keep the share of beneficiaries eligible the same.

The financing package for the MCCA contained a two-tier premium. All beneficiaries would pay a small flat premium, initially set at $6.50 per month. A supplemental income-related premium gradually increased the amount as beneficiaries' tax liabilities increased (effectively a 15 percent surtax on income). The maximum liability was set at $800 annually per enrollee and was imposed on individuals with incomes over $40,000. Couples with incomes over about $70,000 would pay $1,600. Estimates indicated that only about 5 percent of older persons would be subject to these maximum tax levels and that about 40 percent of all the elderly would pay at least some supplemental premium. But the impact of the surtax would rise rapidly over time and affect a larger proportion of Medicare enrollees because it was not indexed for inflation. As peoples' incomes rose each year, the limits would affect a larger share of the population.

The expected impacts of these changes are shown in table 4.1. Overall, Medicare benefits per enrollee were expected to rise by about 7 percent (Christensen and Kasten 1988). New benefits would total about $194, of which $172 would represent reduced cost sharing. Overall, premiums would fully offset these new benefits, averaging $207 per capita. Most beneficiaries would only be liable for a $78 premium increase, however.

Table 4.1. Medicare Benefits Payments, Co-payment Liabilities, and Premiums Payable Per Enrollee Before and After Implementation of Medicare Catastrophic Coverage Act of 1988

	Before	After	Change
Medicare benefit payments per enrollee[a]			
Hospital Insurance	$1,693	$1,747	$54
Supplementary Medical Insurance	1,108	1,91	83
Catastrophic Drug Insurance	0	57	57
Total	2,801	2,995	194
Medicare co-payment liabilities per enrollee			
Hospital Insurance	162	118	−44
Supplementary Medical Insurance	325	262	−63
Catastrophic Drug Insurance	244	179	−65
Total	731	559	−172
Medicare premiums payable per enrollee			
Monthly premiums	290	368	78
Supplementary premiums	0	129	129
Total	290	497	

Source: U.S. Congressional Budget Office (1988).
Note: Table shows effects of Medicare only.
[a] About 22 percent of enrollees were estimated to be entitled to higher Medicare benefit payments under the MCA when fully implemented. This reflects an unduplicated count of those affected by the Hospital Insurance provisions (4 percent), the Supplementary Medical Insurance co-payment cap (7 percent), and the drug provisions (16.8 percent).

So most beneficiaries (about 70 percent) would have gained from the legislation (CBO 1988).

Another important element of the financing, however, was that the premiums were set to begin in 1989, while several of the key benefits were not scheduled to begin until later. Revenues would be considerably higher than outlays in the early years to allow for the buildup of reserves in a newly created trust fund. This feature also had the short-run effect of reducing the federal deficit and would later come under fire by beneficiaries suspicious of whether they were being taxed for new benefits or to pay for deficit reduction.

Winners and Losers

Proponents of the legislation believed they had achieved a major improvement in benefits. For example, the largest interest group representing the elderly, the AARP, enjoyed accolades concerning the important role the organization had played in working with Congress

(Torres-Gil 1989). Other organizations of the elderly and organized labor had also worked hard to secure passage.

The MCCA also had vehement opponents. The drug industry, fearing government interference in its activities, bitterly fought inclusion of the drug benefit in the program. Although the industry could not block the legislation, it managed to water down the drug benefit provisions. For example, the legislation made no reference to any type of cost controls on drugs; instead, the final bill called for beneficiaries to pay higher premiums over time if costs exceeded expectations. The Pharmaceutical Manufacturers Association reportedly spent several million dollars opposing the legislation and seeking limitations on controls over costs (Rich 1987).

The National Committee to Preserve Social Security and Medicare, a latecomer to the debate, was also against the bill, and sought to derail the financing scheme and eliminate the supplemental premium. They mounted a major lobbying and letter-writing campaign that was unsuccessful, at least in part because members of Congress viewed their often deceptive mail campaigns more as a fundraising ploy than legitimate grassroots organizing (Simon 1989). Opposition to the legislation from other seniors' groups was only beginning to get organized when the legislation passed.

As table 4.1 shows, there were clearly individual winners and losers even though the overall impact was essentially budget neutral. On the benefit side, additional benefits directed at low-income beneficiaries through the Medicaid program ensured that many low-income enrollees would be winners. Because various groups used different amounts of health services, the level of benefits received would have varied in any given year. For example, the very old with high rates of hospital use were more likely to benefit than younger, healthier enrollees.

Many opponents of the legislation pointed out that few people would directly receive help in any given year and thus, the MCCA was a "bad deal." They ignored the fact that everyone with the new coverage was at risk and would gain needed protection whether or not they actually used it in any one year. This is the principle of catastrophic coverage, often ignored when people focus on winners and losers.

Repeal

Criticism of the MCCA made it clear that beneficiaries as a group either did not understand the fundamental principle of catastrophic insurance or did not value such protection very highly. Even after the MCCA passed in 1988, opponents—led by the Pharmaceutical Manufacturers Association and the National Committee to Preserve Social Security and Medicare—kept up a steady barrage of protest and captured considerable media attention.

Two contradictory sets of information fed this opposition. First came word in the spring of 1989 that the U.S. Treasury expected tax collections from the supplemental premium on the elderly to be higher than anticipated, generating a considerable buildup in the catastrophic coverage trust fund. This again fueled concerns that the new legislation was deliberately aimed at reducing the deficit at the expense of the elderly.

But then, the Congressional Budget Office released a new set of estimates indicating that the costs of some benefits had been severely underestimated. In particular, improvements in the SNF benefit were projected to cost more than six times the original estimate. In addition, re-estimates of the costs of the drug benefit using newly available data proved twice as high as the original figure (CBO 1989a). These new estimates indicated that the full supplemental premium would be needed over time.

Although some of the interest groups, such as the National Committee to Preserve Social Security and Medicare, argued to keep all the benefits while changing the financing, most of the initial debate centered on what benefits could be retained if the supplemental premium were eliminated. There was little serious discussion of adding additional revenue sources: the original agreement to stick with a self-financed benefit package remained intact. The difficulty lay in deciding which benefits were the most important. Each had proponents who had worked within the legislative framework during passage and who felt they had already compromised enough.

Many options were proposed, but none captured the imagination of enough members of Congress to go anywhere. On October 4, 1989, the House of Representatives voted to repeal all of the MCCA except the Medicaid provisions. In the early hours of November 22, 1989, after several last ditch attempts to find a compromise before adjournment, Congress took the nearly unprecedented step of repealing a major piece of social legislation only one year after passage and before most benefits had been implemented.

Lessons from the MCCA

The unusual step of quickly repealing major legislation highlights important policy lessons, some of which can be seen in the 2003 legislative effort. Beneficiaries objected to the supplemental premium more than any other element of the legislation. Medicare's Part B premium had always been a flat payment assessed on everyone except the very poorest beneficiaries. The new financing was a dramatic departure.

Although only a small share of beneficiaries—about 5 percent—would actually have had to pay the maximum supplemental amount, much of the publicity generated by groups supporting repeal suggested otherwise. For example, one flyer produced by a group calling itself the Seniors' Coalition Against the Tax asked in bold letters: "Will you get an $800 tax bill for catastrophic coverage this year?" Its readers were not invited to think there might be more than one answer. Pharmaceutical companies used this discomfort to help stimulate opposition to a drug plan they feared. In fact, these companies helped to finance some of the "grass roots" consumer opposition.

Throughout the debate, both Congress and the organizations supporting the legislation took care to retain the nomenclature of supplemental premiums to distinguish it from a "tax." But it was to be collected by the IRS through the regular income tax structure and calculated based on how much income tax a beneficiary owed, just like a surtax.

The final MCCA legislation offered net benefit increases to a majority of Medicare beneficiaries. But these were typically modest and came in a bewildering variety of forms. There was no consistent theme or logic to the many disparate changes in the MCCA, making the whole somehow seem less than the sum of its parts. Further, catastrophic coverage itself can be a hard sell because, by definition, only a small proportion of enrollees will use the benefits. Finally, many who would have paid the income surtax already had these protections through employer-subsidized plans. Health policy experts agreed that the MCCA provisions were needed additions to the Medicare package, especially the additions that provided protection to persons facing the danger of financial catastrophe from high out-of-pocket costs. But the average beneficiary simply did not see it that way.

THE PRESCRIPTION DRUG, IMPROVEMENT, AND MODERNIZATION ACT

After considerable controversy, Congress passed the Medicare Prescription Drug, Improvement, and Modernization Act (MMA) in November 2003, and President Bush signed it into law in December 2003, providing the largest benefit expansion in the program's history along with major changes to the program structure. A number of issues remain controversial, however. As passed, this legislation was expected to increase federal spending by $395 billion through 2013. The drug benefit itself was expected to cost slightly more: $410 billion over 10 years (CBO 2003). In 2004, however, information from the administration was released that suggested the overall costs would be much higher—$534 billion (Holtz-Eakin 2004). Even at this level of spending, funding constraints have resulted in a standard package that creates a gap in coverage for persons in the middle range of spending on prescription drugs. The adequacy of the drug benefit and the details of its structure constitute two major areas of continuing controversy. Aside from the addition of a drug benefit, the legislation also significantly changed the basic Medicare program that will affect beneficiaries both directly and indirectly. Among the most controversial of these changes is how much the emphasis on private plans puts beneficiaries in traditional Medicare at a disadvantage. And, while the low-income protections in the legislation are a substantial improvement over the House and Senate bills, the legislation still excludes a number of Medicare beneficiaries who need help and imposes a substantial burden on states to help fund these low-income benefits. Since important pieces of the legislation did not go into effect until 2006 and hence are just under way, the ultimate impacts are yet to be seen.

The details of the drug benefit's structure, including reliance on private standalone plans, consumer fallback protections, and preclusion of private fill-in benefits, will likely create problems for beneficiaries. Although in many cases these issues seem to be small pieces of the overall law, these and related provisions will determine how well this new legislation will operate.

In tying a drug benefit to broader changes in Medicare, the MMA also creates changes that supporters claim will help reduce the growth of spending over time and determine whether traditional Medicare will remain a viable option. In effect, the MMA promotes the expansion of private options for covering Medicare benefits on the belief that competition and the private sector will achieve long-term savings for the program. The traditional part of Medicare is basically left as it is. Republican supporters, the Bush Administration, and even the AARP have argued that these improvements will not hurt the traditional fee-for-service portion of the program. But even its supporters recognized it was necessary to offer a drug benefit to make other, less popular reforms promoting private plans more palatable to beneficiaries.

The basic tenet of these reforms is the creation of an expanded role for the private sector, with the implicit goal of eventually replacing or limiting participation in the traditional Medicare option (in which the government bears the risk and individuals are free to go to most doctors, hospitals, and other care providers). In addition to retaining a role for the Medicare + Choice managed care plans, the new law encourages participation of preferred provider organizations (PPOs) and combines both in a new option, Medicare Advantage. Strong financial incentives are created to attract new private plans to the program. Payment levels are initially very generous before they transition to a negotiated price system in 2007. In 2010, a demonstration in six areas will be undertaken, moving toward a defined contribution approach in which traditional Medicare will be substantially changed so as to operate as simply another plan option. A defined contribution approach essentially offers a fixed dollar amount that is not tied to the true costs of insurance. This essentially shifts risks from the government to individuals. And since individuals are generally not able to negotiate premium costs, critics worry that too much power will shift to private plans. Such an approach is very controversial and has been examined at length elsewhere. (See, for example, American Academy of Actuaries 2002; Christianson, Parente, and Taylor 2002.) The next chapter focuses more on how the immediate changes to increase Medicare privatization will affect beneficiaries and whether this approach will generate savings for the program.

Adequacy of the Drug Benefit

Budget constraints and the voluntary nature of the prescription drug benefit largely determined how the benefit would need to be designed. Likely remembering the MCCA, Congress did not wish to make the benefit mandatory since some beneficiaries already had good coverage. To attract participants to a voluntary program, Congress had to offer some benefits to those with low levels of prescription drug spending or otherwise healthy beneficiaries would be less likely to enroll. Moreover, there was also a goal of providing protection from catastrophic expenses for those with high levels of spending even though MCCA proved that beneficiaries undervalue benefits that only provide catastrophic protection. But because the Congress wanted to control how much the drug benefit would cost, the basic coverage had to be limited. Essentially, offering coverage at the low end of the spending scale and for catastrophic coverage left a gap in the middle. Thus, the legislation creates a gap, or "doughnut hole," in coverage. The desire to hold down the costs of the benefit also limited how far up the income scale protections for the low-income population could go—setting that limit at 150 percent of the federal poverty line.

The Gap. The standard benefit established in the legislation creates a gap in coverage between $2,250 and $5,100 in total spending. This comes after beneficiaries pay a $250 deductible and then 25 percent of the next $2,000 in total spending. At that point, the beneficiary will have spent $750 out of pocket. Before the catastrophic portion of the benefit begins, each individual must pay $3,600 out of pocket. In this way, the next $2,850 in spending on drugs must come from the beneficiary or his family.[4] When that requirement is met at $5,100 in total spending on drugs, the plan will cover 95 percent of additional spending. As a result, the average share of spending the government covers will vary depending on beneficiaries' total drug costs. Figure 4.1 shows the average percentage covered by a standard plan at various spending levels. The share paid by the plan reaches a high point at $2,250, declines until $5,100, and then rises again. So the coverage gap for the basic drug benefit arises just where the growth in spending on drugs is occurring for persons with chronic conditions. It is exactly in this range where better coverage of drugs for the chronically ill could ultimately help to lower health care spending elsewhere. Ironically, the government's share of the costs for someone with $5,000 in spending is 32 percent—less than half the share paid for someone with just $2,000 in drug expenditures (65 percent).

Forty-four percent of Medicare beneficiaries are projected to have drug expenses in 2006 of more than $2,250, taking them into the coverage gap (figure 4.2). While nearly a third of that group would ultimately receive catastrophic protection, the gap in coverage would still affect them.[5]

Figure 4.1. Beneficiary and Government Share of Spending in 2006, at Individual Expenditure Levels, under the New Medicare Drug Benefit

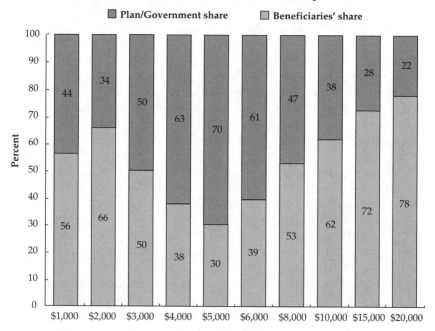

Individual's total annual drug expenditures

Source: Author's calculations.

Figure 4.2. Medicare Population by Level of Prescription Drug Spending

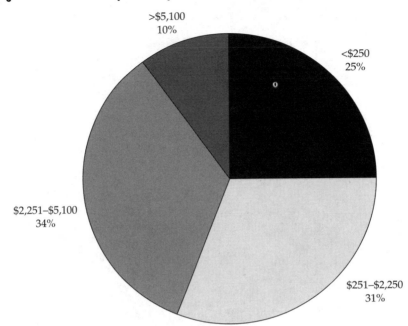

Source: CBO (2004).
Note: These figures represent the spending distribution for all beneficiaries. The distribution for those who participate in the program or who receive low income subsidies may vary.

Beneficiaries with chronic conditions are particularly likely to have drug expenses in the range of $3,000 to $5,000. Figure 4.3 shows the share of beneficiaries by number of chronic conditions. As indicated, a large proportion of Medicare beneficiaries have two or more chronic conditions and these conditions are strongly correlated to high spending on prescription drugs (table 4.2). Many take several drugs every day, each of which can cost $1,000 or more a year.

Many discussions about the gap report it as being smaller than it is because the rules for coverage are established on two different bases. Initially, the deductible and co-payments are tied to total spending. But eligibility for catastrophic protection is linked to out-of-pocket spending. Why does this matter? Essentially, it restricts the ability of any drug plan to fill in the gap in the benefit package. That is, only contributions from the individual, the family, or a state pharmaceutical benefit program count toward the out-of-pocket spending requirement.

While the new law will allow plans the flexibility to vary the deductible and co-pay structure, the $3,600 out-of-pocket requirement remains the same. If a private insurance plan covers spending above $2,250,

Figure 4.3. Distribution of Medicare Beneficiaries by Number of Chronic Conditions

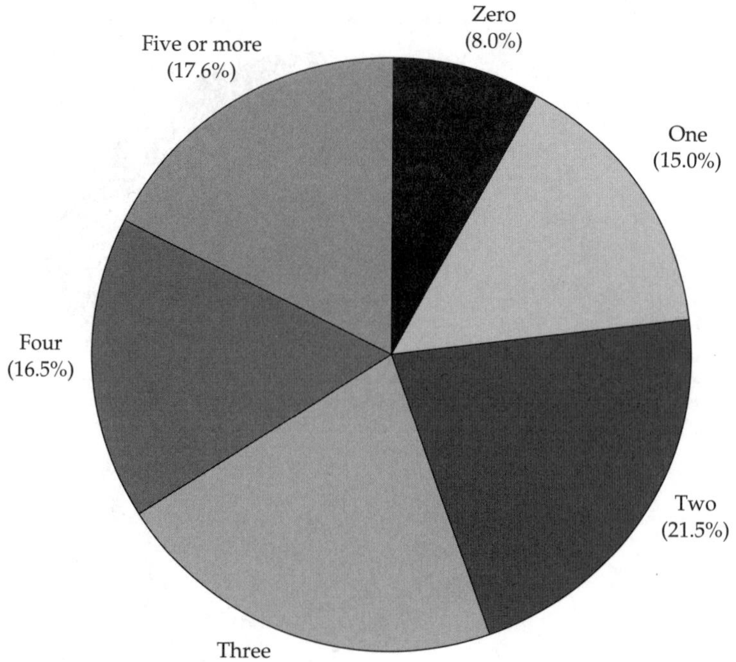

Source: Boccuti, Moon, and Dowling (2003).
Note: Excludes facility beneficiaries.

the gap would not be reduced; rather, it would just begin at a higher spending level. For example, if a private insurance company sold a policy to pay 100 percent of the spending between $2,250 and $4,250, then the catastrophic protection would not begin until $7,100 in total spending—the point at which the individual would have spent $3,600 out of pocket. This is quite different from how supplemental policies work under the rest of Medicare, where the government does not have any stake in who pays the deductibles and co-payments.

The rationale for such heavy discouragement of gap-filling is that if individuals purchased more comprehensive supplemental benefits, the cost of the catastrophic protections would rise. That is, more people would "make it" to the catastrophic spending level ($5,100) if they had such coverage. This can be viewed two ways: people will be discouraged from using drugs unnecessarily, or people in need of help (who limit drug use since they cannot afford it) may never spend enough

Table 4.2. Annual Prescription Fills and Average Drug Spending, by Number of Chronic Conditions

Number of chronic conditions	Prescription fills	Average drug spending (2006 dollars)	Percentage with more than $2,000 in drug spending (%)
0	8	1,346	18
1	12	1,819	27
2	18	2,543	43
3	24	3,426	56
4	30	4,046	66
5 or more	40	5,673	75
Total	23	3,320	51

Source: Boccuti, Moon, and Dowling (2003).

Notes: Excludes end-stage renal disease and beneficiaries living in a nursing facility. Spending in 2006 adjusted for Congressional Budget Office estimates.

out of pocket to reach the catastrophic level. In practice, some of both of these responses would likely occur.

Further, since this is a voluntary benefit, sweetening the coverage for those with higher spending and lessening it for those with more limited drug spending would result in adverse selection. Until or unless a very good risk selection adjuster is established, plans may be reluctant to experiment in this way. The government offers some risk protections to plans, but only time will tell whether that will be sufficient to encourage plans to risk a change in the basic benefit structure.

This part of the legislation is vulnerable to attack when beneficiaries understand these rules. They may perceive inequities in providing better protections to those with $2,000 in spending than those with $5,000 in spending (as a share of their burdens). Filling the gap without changing other coverage would be expensive, however, since over 40 percent of all beneficiaries in 2006 will have expenditures greater than $2,250.

Low-Income Provisions. For persons who qualify for low-income protection, this legislation generally improves drug coverage. For incomes up to 135 percent of the federal poverty level, beneficiaries will pay no premium and be subject to only small co-payments of $2 per generic and $5 per brand-name drug (subsidy level A).[6] This would be less generous for individuals covered by Medicaid in the approximately 16 states that provide comprehensive benefits and lower or no co-payments. But many individuals would potentially be newly eligible for drug benefits since the standard eligibility level for Medicaid is 74 percent of the poverty level, and only 17 states cover Medicare eligibles up to 100 percent of the poverty level. Between 135 and 150 percent of the poverty level, the benefits phase out as a sliding scale premium is charged, a $50 deductible is added, and co-payments are increased (subsidy level B). The CBO has estimated that of the 14.7 million Medicare beneficiaries who would be eligible for the low-income subsidies, 6.2 million are dual eligibles (table 4.3). So over half of this group would be newly eligible for a drug benefit.[7]

Above 150 percent of the poverty level, the benefit is the same for everyone and individuals with incomes slightly higher than the 150 percent cutoff would find it difficult to pay the premium and required cost-sharing for a drug benefit. For example, someone spending $3,000 on drugs would pay about 12 percent of his or her annual income out of pocket even if they purchased the coverage.[8] Others in this group may end up no better off than at present if they decide they cannot afford the premiums. In such a case, they would likely continue underusing the drugs they need.

The legislation also relies on asset tests to limit eligibility for low-income protections. Assets exclude the value of the home and mainly capture financial resources. Nonetheless, these are restrictive limits. For persons with incomes below 135 percent of the poverty level, the asset test is set at $6,000 per single and $9,000 per couple. Further, many low-income beneficiaries are likely to be excluded from these programs because of the complexity of the qualification process. For those with incomes between 135 and 150 percent of the poverty level, the asset tests are less stringent (at $10,000 for individuals and $20,000 for couples) and an expedited form will be used. (In addition, persons with incomes below 135 percent of poverty but whose assets fall between the limits can qualify for the less generous subsidies.) But even these higher asset-test cutoffs are quite stringent, especially considering

Table 4.3. Eligibility of Medicare Beneficiaries in 2006 for Low-Income Subsidies

	Income (% of federal poverty level)				
	Below 100%	101%–135%	136%–150%	151% and above	Total
	Number of eligible beneficiaries (millions)				
Subsidy A					
Dual eligibles	4.4	1.1	0.2	0.6	6.4
All other beneficiaries	2.7	3.1	0.0	0.0	.8
Subsidy B	0.2	0.5	1.2	0.0	1.9
Not eligible for low-income subsidies	0.4	0.9	0.5	23.7	25.4
Total Medicare beneficiaries	**7.7**	**5.6**	**1.8**	**24.2**	**39.4**

Source: Adapted from CBO (2004).

that beneficiaries are likely to have planned to stretch their modest savings over many years to supplement their incomes (Moon, Friedland, and Shirey 2002). The CBO estimated that 1.8 million individuals who would be income eligible for benefits would be excluded entirely by the asset test, and another 0.7 million would receive lower subsidies because they would not meet the lower asset-test requirement (table 4.3).

The combination of requiring strict income and asset tests and the reluctance of many Medicare beneficiaries to identify themselves as "poor" is expected to hold down the number of Medicare beneficiaries participating in the subsidized drug benefit (Summer and Friedland 2002). For example, in calculating the likely costs of the legislation, the Congressional Budget Office assumed that only 75 percent of those with incomes below 135 percent of the poverty level would participate and just 35 percent of those with incomes between 135 percent and 150 percent of the poverty level would do so (CBO 2003). These shares are similar to those found for participation in the current Medicare savings programs.

Will states do more to fill in these gaps in low-income protections? First, states are precluded from filling in the co-pays required in the legislation from individuals with incomes below 135 percent of the poverty level. States are allowed to use funds from a prescription drug benefit program to fill in the larger gaps in the basic benefit. And several of the larger state programs might continue to aid people with incomes above 150 percent of the poverty level, for example. Such aid will count toward the out-of-pocket spending requirement (and hence provide improved protection for beneficiaries), but states receive no matching funds for this effort. Further, the legislation also requires that states continue to pay a substantial amount of their current costs of covering the dual eligibles through a provision referred to as the "clawback." The legislation calls for the contribution to decline from 90 percent of what the expenses would have been without the Medicare drug benefit in 2006 to 75 percent of that level by 2015 and beyond. The state contributions will also be adjusted upward to reflect increases in the number of dually eligible individuals. Some states may actually end up owing more to the federal government than they would have spent on their own. Particularly in the early years, when the requirements for contributions are high, states facing budget problems are unlikely to seek new ways to expand spending on the Medicare population.

Indexation of the Benefit Structure. Finally, the various cutoffs for the drug benefit, including the gap, would be indexed by the annual increase in the cost of the drug benefit itself. As a consequence, the $3,600 gap is expected to rise to $6,400 in 2013—a 78 percent increase (table 4.4). So, in 2013, catastrophic protection will not begin until an individual has spent $9,066 on prescription drugs. Yet eligibility for low-income protection and the incomes of Medicare beneficiaries are expected to rise at a much slower rate over that time period—by about half that amount. If that is the case, the share of income that beneficiaries devote to drugs will rise, even for those enrolled in the drug benefit. For example, a person with income just above 150 percent of the poverty level spending 12 percent of her income on drugs and the drug premium for coverage in 2006 would spend about 18 percent of her income on drugs and the premium by 2013.

The Structure of the Drug Benefit

The new law only allows drug benefits to be offered through private insurers (unless a fall-back plan is needed), thereby creating a more cumbersome system of coverage for beneficiaries who choose to remain in traditional Medicare. In fact, no additional benefits would be added to the traditional Medicare program, so most beneficiaries would retain their supplemental policies to fill in those gaps. Consequently, many beneficiaries would likely have to purchase two private supplemental policies in addition to Medicare—a Medigap plan and a drug plan. Those who now have Medigap plans with a drug benefit would need to enroll in a new plan (or retain their old one without the drug coverage). Since the new plans are subsidized, they will represent a better value than buying drugs through Medigap, although many beneficiaries will still likely be confused about what to do. Each year, this group will have to make tough decisions, perhaps buying a less comprehensive Medigap policy if the costs of the drug plans rise steeply, for example. Beneficiaries also will need to compare the costs of traditional Medicare plus two supplemental plans with the more comprehensive but potentially restrictive private options to make appropriate decisions. Medicare beneficiaries with employer-

Table 4.4. Standard Drug Benefit, 2006 and 2013

	2006	2013
Annual deductible	$250	$445
Coinsurance to initial limit	25%	25%
Initial limit	$2,250	$4,000
Out-of-pocket threshold	$3,600	$6,400
Coverage gap	$2,850	$5,066
Coinsurance about OOP (greater of)	$2/$5 or 5%	$3/$8 or 5%

Source: Adapted from Congressional Budget Office (2004).

subsidized retiree plans are also likely face new decisions when employers change their plans.

In addition, other aspects of the structure of the benefits may be problematic for individuals, causing disruption over time and new complexities added by rules on which specific drugs will be covered.

Fall-Back Plans. In part because of the geographic variations in spending on prescription drugs, it was feared that some regions may not be attractive to private drug plans. In that case, fall-back provisions are critical to ensure that beneficiaries in traditional Medicare have access to drug coverage. The new legislation will create a federal government–run drug plan in areas where less than two private plans participate (only one of which must be a stand-alone drug benefit). The government would bear the risk and contract with a pharmacy benefit management company or some other entity to process claims and administer the program. The fall-back will remain in place only until new private plans enter the market.

Moreover, the rules established for fall-back plans do not allow the government to take advantage of the fact that a fall-back plan would have lower administrative costs than a stand-alone drug plan. That is, the legislation explicitly requires that the government must use the average administrative costs for private plans in setting the fall-back premium.

Although a number of problems could arise from this approach, the initial offerings by private plans have set aside the need for fall back options—at least for now. Indeed, in the fall of 2005, beneficiaries in every state faced choices of at least 40 different options. In some cases, companies offered multiple options to potential enrollees, reflecting different levels of comprehensiveness of plans—for example eliminating the initial deductible. These plans also offered a wide range of premiums and formulary rules.

Delayed Sign-Up. Substantial financial penalties will be assessed on beneficiaries who delay enrollment past the initial period. At a minimum, the premium will increase by 1 percent for each month delay in enrollment. It could be higher if the Secretary of Health and Human Services certifies that actuarial costs are greater. Another confusing aspect of this penalty is when it applies to persons who have drug coverage from other sources. No penalty applies if that coverage is as good as or better than the Medicare benefit. If, however, such coverage is not as good (i.e., it is not "creditable"), then a penalty would apply if and when a beneficiary seeks to switch to a Medicare plan. Information on creditable coverage may be another source of confusion.

To protect beneficiaries, plans need to balance mechanisms used to encourage people to sign up against penalties for those who may be skeptical or confused about the benefits, especially in the plans' early years. A longer initial sign-up period before the assessment of penalties would improve this problem. As of December 2005, only about 1 million of the potential 20 million beneficiaries who may choose to join stand-alone drug plans had signed up, reflecting at least in part the massive confusion that the large number of available options created (Pear 2005).

Formularies. Formularies, which specify the drugs a plan covers, will likely be a major source of cost-containment efforts. For example, within a therapeutic class of drugs aimed at meeting particular needs (such as lowering cholesterol), plans can limit the number of drugs covered to just two. The offerings in the fall of 2005 have generally been inclusive in terms of their formularies, but have relied upon a range of other restrictions that as yet are not fully understood. For example, plans can specify different levels of co-payments by type of drug, differentiating between preferred drugs and others within a therapeutic category. Plans are also promoting generic over brandname drugs. Some are requiring "step therapy" in which less powerful drugs are used before stepping up to more powerful ones, or other forms of prior authorization. These tools can reduce the costs of drugs and hence lower beneficiary premiums. But they also add to the confusion, can change, and do not have to be disclosed before people enroll in a particular drug plan. That is, the legislation indicates that the formulary only needs to be disclosed at time of enrollment, and even then, beneficiaries may only be given a web site or phone number to obtain that information.

Generally, pharmacy benefit management firms (PBMs) or other entities which offer drug plans steer patients to drugs for which the manufacturer has offered the biggest discount. But this establishes economic screens for choosing drugs that may not be the best way to approach formularies. For example, without good knowledge and information about the comparative effectiveness and presence of side effects of drugs within a therapeutic category, patients may not be steered in the manner that best meets their health needs. Thus, a plan may not offer a drug that has the lowest side effects or works best for some patients. The legislation gives plans considerable latitude for structuring formularies. Some plans may be very restrictive to obtain the lowest prices and hence keep their premiums low. Other plans may offer more drugs within a particular category and attract enrollees on the claim of a more comprehensive (and expensive) benefit.

The Veterans Administration and a number of states have begun to modify their formularies where information on medical effectiveness is available and therefore are not using price as the determining factor. Additional independent information and protections of this type are needed for a high quality benefit. Medicare could help advance knowledge in this area if even modest resources (compared with the costs of the drug plan) were invested. The MMA did not fund such efforts, however.

Stand-Alone Plans and Traditional Medicare. For beneficiaries who choose to get all their benefits from private plans, the proposed drug benefit would be integrated into an overall package. But for those who choose to stay in traditional Medicare, a separate, stand-alone drug plan would provide drug benefits. Many private- and public-sector experts have expressed doubts about insurers' ability to offer stand-alone benefits (Pear 2003). For example, risk adjustment is likely to work better for an integrated benefit package than for a stand-alone benefit. In addition, such a benefit requires its own administrative structure. For these reasons, stand-alone plans likely would be more expensive for insurers to provide than integrated benefits. This could saddle those who remain in traditional Medicare with higher costs.

At least initially, the protections for private plans may encourage insurers to participate. Indeed, in 2006, many different groups are offering plans. With high protections against risk, many insurers, PBMs, pharmacies, and others are participating, perhaps fearing the loss of market share and lost future opportunities if they do not immediately enter the market.

Greater Privatization in Medicare

The 2003 legislation also establishes Medicare Advantage for HMOs, private fee-for-service plans, and, for the first time, preferred provider organizations (PPOs). The MMA also changes the payment structure for private plans, adding new financial incentives for such plans to participate. Supporters of this approach cite the flexibility of private plans to adjust quickly to changes in health care delivery and the new and innovative approaches they may include. These traits compare favorably with the rigidity of Medicare, its "one-size-fits-all" approach, and the extensive regulatory controls on the program. Further, when plans are given a single monthly payment to cover all of a beneficiary's needs, they face strong incentives to coordinate care and provide it efficiently. Proponents and opponents of a private plan approach agree that the Medicare + Choice option failed to serve beneficiaries well. Proponents of managed care criticize the government for its management and oversight of the plans. Managed-care critics cite the higher costs generated by Medicare + Choice that resulted in no savings to the government.

Because so many plans withdrew or cut their offerings, the legislation provides special subsidies to serve as incentives for Medicare Advantage and stand-alone drug plans to participate in Medicare. At the same time, its supporters have touted privatization as the means for achieving slower rates of growth in Medicare spending over time. A second claim is that the new law will not harm traditional Medicare in any way. Skepticism about these claims represents the heart of criticism leveled at the legislation. And concern about the problems arising from risk selection and the lack of a good risk-adjustment mechanism are essential parts of that debate.

The Likelihood of Savings from Relying on Market Forces. Opposition to relying on private plans for Medicare stems from evidence suggesting that these plans are unlikely to slow cost growth over time, and from practical concerns about whether new features, such as stand-alone prescription drug plans, will work at all. To date, the evidence shows that privatization will achieve few, if any, savings for Medicare. Certainly the claim that privatization is essential to holding down Medicare's future costs is on shaky ground. Recent experience with Medicare + Choice plans suggests beneficiaries are paying more out of pocket and getting less value in return (Gold and Achman 2003). Moreover, over the past 30 years, Medicare growth has been below that of private insurance and the Federal Employees Health Benefits Program (Boccuti and Moon 2003).

With private plans serving mainly healthier Medicare beneficiaries, these plans appear to be more efficient than they are once the effects of risk selection are taken into account. This risk selection has resulted in excess payments to plans by the federal government (see the discussion with regard to the BBA in chapter 3). Plans have financed additional benefits for their enrollees with the excess payments, making them appear to be more successful in delivering care efficiently than has actually been the case. In fact, it is difficult for private plans to compete with Medicare on cost grounds. Managed care can obtain discounts from hospitals, doctors, and other care providers to hold down costs, but few plans can do as well as Medicare in that regard. Further, administrative costs for private plans are quite high. The only other avenue is to reduce the use of goods and services. But, so far, most private plans have not created new or innovative delivery systems that generate substantial savings while retaining consumer satisfaction. Rather, they have succeeded largely where they have attracted healthier-than-average enrollees and have implicitly been overpaid. Chapter 5 discusses these issues in more detail.

Under MMA, payments to private plans are likely to continue to exceed what it would cost to provide benefits through the traditional Medicare program. In 2004, for example, payments to private plans exceeded the costs of traditional Medicare, even assuming no risk selection (Biles, Nicholas, and Cooper 2004). The CBO estimated that between 2005 and 2013, private plans would add $14 billion to the costs of the legislation for bonus payments. The subsidies would be direct, through explicitly higher payments to plans, and indirect, since they would include in the monthly payment to plans an implicit subsidy to support medical education and care for indigent hospital patients. These items add to traditional Medicare's costs but are not usually an expense to private plans. Nonetheless, these costs are implicitly built into plan payments.[9]

These higher payments are intended to jumpstart a competitive system, but it is reasonable to ask when such subsidies would pay returns, if ever. Experimenting with new private plans for Medicare makes sense, but private plans should add value either through savings or through new and innovative approaches to care. Otherwise, spending scarce public dollars on such an effort is difficult to justify.

How might private plans save money for Medicare over time? What has to happen to make them less expensive? In the case of PPOs, savings arise from enrolling efficient providers in their networks who are less likely to order tests and procedures. But in addition, savings also come from paying very low amounts on services used outside the network, both by having higher co-payments and by setting the amounts they pay for such services at a very low level.

This creates a conundrum for Medicare. The legislation limits how much beneficiaries must pay for using out-of-network services. But this effectively eliminates a major tool that PPOs rely on for cost savings. There will likely be pressure over time to give PPOs more flexibility in paying for out-of-network services to keep them in the program. But that would put beneficiaries at risk of paying substantially more to go out of network.

Further, the emphasis on consumer choice can undermine plans' ability to generate price competition and savings. If plans can vary in the benefits they offer, they may use marketing and benefit structure, rather than lower premiums, to attract customers. For this reason, some proponents of competition emphasize that cost savings also will depend on how much price is emphasized, and hence the need to ensure plans vary little in terms of what they offer consumers.[10] Ironically, one of the selling points for relying on private plans—that people can get precisely the benefits they want rather than being put into a "one-size-fits-all" structure—may be at odds with holding down the costs of health coverage.

Why should beneficiaries care that substantially lower rates of cost growth are unlikely to occur from the changes the legislation establishes? First, there will likely be greater pressure over time to allow provisions such as high-balance billing on out-of-network use for persons in PPOs to achieve savings. Further, lower-priced plans, even of questionable quality, may be promoted, putting traditional Medicare or higher-priced plans at a disadvantage. The legislature also dictates that plans will face change over time in the way that their payments are established. In 2007, plans are supposed to negotiate rates with the government to generate savings for the Medicare program. At that point, the system will face the same challenges faced after 1997: plans accustomed to receiving extra payments beyond the cost of providing benefits under traditional Medicare will have to cut back on any extra benefits they offer, raise premiums to beneficiaries, or continue to receive extra government subsidies. The first two options could result in a drop-off in enrollment as happened in 1997; the third would lead to a continuation of higher costs for Medicare Advantage than for traditional Medicare.

A Level Playing Field for Medicare? For beneficiaries, the subsidies in Medicare Advantage create an uneven playing field, penalizing beneficiaries in traditional Medicare. That is, thanks to higher payments to the private plans, Medicare Advantage insurers will be able to offer improved benefits, while traditional Medicare will be constrained to its inadequate benefit package. On a per capita basis, the differential amounts to about $550 per beneficiary (Biles et al. 2004). Since individuals unwilling to take a chance on a new insurance option are likely to be sicker than average, this approach favors the healthy over the sick.[11] Medicare Advantage plans also have some additional flexibility in coordinating drug benefits with other coverage. They can create more generous drug benefits, although the catastrophic out-of-pocket spending requirement must still be met.

Moreover, since individuals who wish to remain in traditional Medicare must purchase two separate supplemental policies to obtain comprehensive coverage, the administrative costs that beneficiaries will have to bear and the complexity that arises are likely to also favor individuals moving into the new private options for coverage. Again, this is likely to bias the playing field in favor of private plans. In describing the new PPO options, supporters have tended to suggest that they are just like traditional Medicare in terms of individuals being able to choose any doctor or hospital they wish. This is an optimistic portrayal of PPOs, since going out of network (to get "any" doctor) will likely mean substantially higher costs for beneficiaries. But if "educational" materials over-sell these new plans, beneficiaries may enroll in them with false hopes. Large shifts of beneficiaries to the new PPO options may not be a valid test of private plans versus traditional Medicare under these conditions.

Further Privatization in 2010. The MMA establishes a demonstration under Medicare in 2010 that would effectively move the system toward a defined-contribution approach. That is, federal payments to all options under Medicare, including the traditional part of the program, would be based on a share of the average of the premiums in all

Medicare options. This would place a cap on government's contribution to the cost of the benefit package. As a result, any plan with a bid of higher-than-average cost would have to charge substantially higher premiums from beneficiaries. This could potentially divide Medicare beneficiaries on the basis of their ability to pay higher premiums. Moreover, these higher premiums will not always reflect true differences in benefits or quality of care. Plans that attract a higher-than-average percentage of unhealthy beneficiaries (which will likely include traditional Medicare) will have to charge higher premiums unless a very good risk adjustment mechanism is developed by 2010.

While this would only be a demonstration, individuals in the areas where the demonstration occurs would have no choice. If they are in traditional Medicare and wish to stay there, they will likely face higher premiums over time than their counterparts outside the demonstration areas. In the past, similar demonstrations have been canceled as a result of fervent opposition by both insurers and beneficiaries (Nichols and Reischauer 2000). Thus, it may be difficult to undertake this demonstration since it will potentially harm some beneficiaries relative to others. On the other hand, the temptation may well be to implement this approach fully without having a demonstration. Indeed, limiting payments to private plans (while shifting higher costs onto beneficiaries) may be the only way to ensure that privatization "saves" money.

Other Issues Raised by the Legislation

A wide range of additional issues could be included here. As more details on implementation of the many elements of the MMA become available, additional concerns should undoubtedly be added to the list.

Problems Arising from Complexity. Those who wish to shift their coverage to preferred provider organizations (PPOs) or remain in Medicare HMOs may have most of their needs met in one plan, but they will have to choose among varying benefit packages. In particular, the cost-sharing structures will differ from traditional Medicare and across various plans. The new PPOs the legislation promotes would create in-network and out-of-network benefits, deductibles, and cost sharing, essentially doubling the number of rules for beneficiaries to negotiate. In addition, different PPOs could have different networks of providers, affecting how easy it would be for beneficiaries to find health care services at a reasonable cost. Complicated benefit packages that vary from plan to plan make informed choice extremely difficult. To enable beneficiaries to make true comparisons, standardized benefit designs would be needed. But this would place limits on the flexibility plans could offer.

Information and Support for Decisionmaking. Even well-educated consumers currently struggle to understand Medicare, and substantial numbers of older Americans have either inadequate or marginal health literacy skills. What's more, nearly a quarter of Medicare beneficiaries have health problems such as hearing or cognitive declines that make it difficult to make an informed choice about their care (Moon and Storeygard 2001).

The current level of funding at the Centers for Medicare and Medicaid Services (CMS) for beneficiary education cannot handle the current system, much less meet the greater needs that are arising in the new system. The MMA substantially increased the needs for education and information but provided only modest increases in resources to help beneficiaries make informed choices. New funding of $1 billion has been set aside for all aspects of implementing the new legislation. Yet if half of those resources were devoted to beneficiary information and education, it would only average about $12 per enrollee. Leaving this task to private plans runs the risk of misleading advertising. Beneficiaries require an independent source of information, such as the State Health Insurance Assistance Programs (SHIPs), which offer help to beneficiaries in each state. However, funding would need to be increased substantially to these groups to meet the likely surge of beneficiaries needing help. There was an increase in their budgets for 2005, but that amount was small.

Opportunities for Gaming the System. Complexity in the rules, flexibility of coverage, and other details create opportunities for private plans and providers to game the system. For example, under the Medicare + Choice system, HMOs sometimes denied services to beneficiaries clearly covered by statute. Although knowledgeable case workers were able to straighten out these issues, the same problem often recurred in the same HMO (Medicare Rights Center 2002). At present, there is no way for CMS to learn about recurrent problems of this type since most of the aid provided by SHIPs and other groups have no automatic feedback loop to correct such problems. And not all beneficiaries have access to someone who takes on their case directly. Opportunities for activities such as denial of benefits, arbitrary shifting of drugs on or off the preferred list, and manipulation of payments to out-of-network providers will expand considerably under the new legislation with its new PPOs, stand-alone drug plans, and the bonus program, just to name several areas of likely manipulation. A new Office of Medicare Ombudsman has been created, but limited resources mean that it will largely serve as a clearinghouse to improve and standardize information coming in from a wide variety of sources.

Disruptions over Time. Requirements on private plans—for stand-alone drug benefits and the broader private options—are for one-year commitments. This may create a hardship for beneficiaries, who need a stable source of treatment to reduce confusion and ensure quality of care. If plans are permitted to come in and out of markets, beneficiaries will be faced with the same problems that have caused so much dissatis-faction in Medicare + Choice. In this program, insurers have withdrawn entirely from certain regions. Beneficiaries frequently have to change physicians when joining a new plan, only to repeat the process if it later pulls up stakes or changes its physician network. This can happen even if plans do not withdraw, but instead raise premiums or cut benefits. This may put pressure on beneficiaries to look for a new plan or, as evidence from California suggests, stay in inadequate, expensive plans (Buchmueller 2000). Similar issues are likely to arise for stand-alone drug plans as well as the more comprehensive Medicare Advan-tage plans. Drug plans will be able to change their formularies of covered drugs or alter their provider networks during the course of the year. Strong risk protections and extra payment subsidies for plans in the next few years may encourage many to enter these markets. But beneficiaries may ultimately suffer when requirements change to limit such plan advantages, resulting in a new pattern of withdrawals and benefit cuts. More stability in contracts with private plans ought to be considered, including limitations on how fast premiums can rise and how quickly details of the plan can change.

Increased Part B Deductible in Traditional Medicare. An increase in the Part B deductible has been discussed frequently as a means of saving federal dollars. The MMA indexed the Part B deductible, causing it to rise over time. The $100 deductible has recently been raised to $124 in 2006 and remains low relative to other insurance plans for workers. But other areas of cost-sharing are much higher under Medi-care. The Part B deductible increase that will occur over time now that it is indexed to the cost of Part B makes sense as a structural change, but this change would be better used to reduce cost-sharing in areas where it is too high.

Means-Testing the Part B Premium. The MMA creates a higher Part B premium starting with individuals whose annual incomes exceed $80,000 and couples with incomes above $160,000. Replacing a much more controversial proposal to relate the benefit to income, this require-ment keeps the income test on the revenue side—an important improvement. The CBO estimated that when this provision begins in 2007, it will affect only 3 percent of beneficiaries. The share of benefici-aries subject to the income-related premium is expected to rise to 6 percent by 2013 (CBO 2003).

The payroll taxes that make up about half of Medicare's financing are charged on all wages, no matter how high. As a result, individuals with very high incomes already contribute far more than it costs to serve them. Since the drug benefit is paid out of general revenues, persons with substantial incomes who become Medicare beneficiaries will continue to contribute even after retirement. This new requirement for an income-related premium builds on a financing system that asks higher-income beneficiaries to pay more. Nonetheless, it remains a controversial piece to many supporters of social insurance who see this as a first step toward breaking down the universality of the benefit. When this change was added in the 1988 MCCA, it raised much more controversy than when it was included in the 2003 legislation.

The issue of greatest concern, however, is whether the resources that will be obtained through this mechanism will be substantial enough to justify the considerable new administrative costs and reporting requirements. The Social Security Administration will be required to obtain data from the Internal Revenue Service to establish what premium to charge for each Medicare beneficiary. The information will be based on the prior year's tax return, adjusting as needed for those whose circumstances have changed.

A New Measure of Medicare Financial Health. The prescription drug legislation also created a new measure of Medicare's financial health. Although there has been little discussion about this measure either before or after passage, it will likely have important consequences both for other parts of the legislation and for Medicare's future. While it is not clear whether requirements to respond to this measure will result in further policy changes, history indicates that just sounding alarms about Medicare's financial health can induce policy changes. For example, Oberlander (2003) points out the strong historical relationship between earlier notices that the Part A Trust Fund was in trouble and legislation cutting spending on Medicare. Consequently, it is important to be aware of the flaws in this measure that make it a problematic indicator of Medicare's financial status.

This measure will summarize for each fiscal year the amount of general revenue funds used to finance Medicare as a share of total spending on the program. If, in looking ahead for the current and next six fiscal years, general revenue funding (mainly the federal personal income tax) exceeds 45 percent of Medicare's spending, the trustees are required to issue a funding warning indicating that the program will require "excess general revenue funding." If a warning is given for two consecutive years, a set of required responses from the president and the Congress are triggered in which legislation to deal with excess general revenues is supposed to be introduced.

Why focus only on general revenues? Since they only capture part of all spending on Medicare, they are not necessarily a good indicator of whether spending is too high. Moreover, general revenue contributions to the Medicare program have been part of its funding since the program began. And that share has risen over time for two major reasons: the shift of services to Part B and relief given to beneficiaries from the heavy burdens that the original premium formula created. The first of these reflects improvement in health care delivery; further, it reduced the need for payroll tax increases that otherwise would have been needed for Part A. The second was a policy choice debated and enacted by multiple sessions of Congress in the 1970s and 1980s. Further, as the new prescription drug benefit begins, general revenue contributions will rise substantially. From 2005 to 2006, the share will increase by 7 percentage points, taking the share to 43 percent. As enrollment in the prescription drug program rises or as drug use goes up when low-income beneficiaries have better access to drugs, supporters of the new legislation will find this a desirable consequence. But increased enrollment in the drug plan will inevitably trigger the excess funding warning within just two or three years of the start of the drug program. With current projections, an excess funding warning will probably occur in 2006 or 2007 (Boards of Trustees 2005).

This measure dictates the following likely policy choices: increase the payroll tax—an action often criticized as hurting employment over time—or adopt changes that would directly disadvantage beneficiaries by assessing higher premiums (either flat or income-related) or reducing benefits. Ironically, the direct result may be to cut back on the prescription drug benefit.

LOOKING FORWARD

An interesting contrast emerges between the MCCA and the MMA. Differences reflect both changing times and people's greater willingness to accept more legislative changes in 2003 than in 1988. For example, the MMA's income-related premium caused much less initial stir than did the tax on Medicare beneficiaries established in the catastrophic legislation, even though they have similar impacts. Further, the emphasis on private plans is an approach entirely different from the one taken in 1988. But it is also important to note that after the MCCA passed in 1988, opposition was not highly organized or vocal. Only a year later, when implementation began, did people take notice and express their displeasure.

Will the same thing happen with the MMA? It seems less likely for several reasons. First, the overall package in 1988 was essentially fully covered by higher Part B premiums and the tax on beneficiaries with higher incomes. In 2003, Congress sweetened the package with over $400 billion in new spending out of general revenue. And while a substantial share of beneficiaries will deem the drug benefit inadequate, low-income individuals will be much better off if they participate. Further, the benefit is voluntary and individuals will not have to participate if they wish to forego the coverage (although higher-income persons will have to pay the income-related premium since it is assessed on Part B). This should cause less concern among those with retiree coverage (although the issue of private companies potentially pulling back their coverage is likely to raise considerable concern). Finally, drug company opposition helped to fuel and fund the dissent in 1989. By contrast, as many observers have pointed out about the 2003 legislation, drug companies were able to get much of what they asked for in terms of guarantees against government interference, for example. So they did not oppose the legislation in the same way.

It is difficult to determine how much better off beneficiaries will be over time as a result of the MMA. Although there are substantial subsidies in the drug coverage, the drug benefits will not grow with beneficiaries' needs, and other changes that prove to be unworkable or that place some beneficiaries at risk will create offsetting costs. Further legislation and careful development of regulations could certainly mitigate a number of these issues. However, it may be difficult to engage in a constructive debate on the problems with the legislation after the rancor of the debate over passage and given the sensitivity to the high expected costs of this less-than-comprehensive legislation.

Although many parts of the legislation are just now being brought online, the changes that began in 2004 offer initial lessons. For example, the discount cards made available in 2004 attracted fewer beneficiaries than expected. The complexity of the choices was one barrier—one that holds crucial warnings for implementing the full benefit in 2006. Further, the geographic regions announced at the end of 2004 are likely to create opportunities and barriers for private plans that will need to be closely watched. In the spring of 2005, new estimates of the cost of the drug benefit were released, and although the costs for specific years changed little, considerable attention was paid to the higher costs— resulting from estimates based on 10 years of benefits (2006–2015) rather than the eight-year window offered when the legislation passed (2006–2013).

And the initial response to the prescription drug plan details and open enrollment has been troubling. Large numbers of beneficiaries have been confused by the plans and seem to be delaying any decision to enroll (Pear 2005). Moreover, the automatic enrollment process for transferring dual eligibles from Medicaid drug coverage to private plans also seems to hold the potential for substantial problems (Nemore 2005). It remains to be seen whether this drug benefit will be counted as a success by the end of 2006.

The MMA put in place four key themes that will emerge as Medicare's future unfolds; these themes will be the subject of the next three chapters. The first is the role that private plans will play compared with traditional Medicare. As noted above, the unlevel playing field the legislation perpetuated gives private plans an advantage over traditional Medicare, at least for the foreseeable future. The confidence placed in private plans reflects more the faith of legislators than any evidence on advantages that private plans might be able to offer compared with traditional Medicare. The debate over the appropriate structure for the Medicare program will be addressed in chapter 5.

The inadequacies of the drug benefit, already under discussion, generated attention at the end of 2005 when the plans were announced. The adequacy of Medicare's overall benefit package will also be discussed as well as whether the inefficient and complex system of supplementary insurance for those who remain in traditional Medicare will continue. Chapter 6 examines those issues and possible improvements.

The third and fourth themes that stem from the MMA are financing issues. With little discussion or debate, the decision was to fund the new drug benefit almost solely from general revenues. This will accelerate a longstanding trend of supporting a larger share of Medicare from general revenues. Since Part B of the program has risen faster than Part A—largely as a result of changes in the way health care is delivered in the United States—general revenues make up a larger share of Medicare than in the past.

Ironically, however, the fourth theme contradicts the third by challenging the desirability of using general revenues to fund Medicare. Under the heading of "cost containment," the MMA creates a rule that will raise alarms when the share of general revenue financing Medicare reaches 45 percent. The impetus will be on the president and Congress to do something to fix this "problem." But the "problem" is linked directly to the decision to fund the drug benefit out of general revenues. The unwillingness of legislators to take on a financing debate for Medicare is likely the reason these contradictory themes are found in one piece of legislation. As a result, this catch-22 means a near-certain financing crisis in the next several years. These two financing issues will be considered together in chapter 7.

5

ARE PRIVATE PLANS THE ANSWER FOR MEDICARE?

Over the past four decades, Medicare has remained primarily an indemnity-based insurance program, with the government serving as the insurer and paying on a fee-for-service basis. The pressures of financing over the past 25 years have resulted in many incremental changes to the program, usually on reforming payment systems for various providers of care and on restraining growth in these payments. But, in part because past changes already have pared back payment levels to providers of services and kept the comprehensiveness of coverage limited, many policymakers are now looking for more dramatic approaches to hold down long-term costs as the baby boom generation approaches eligibility age.

The current "magic bullet" that has captured the imagination of many is reliance on private insurance to help curb spending costs.[1] This approach would presumably result in greater efficiency stemming from relying on competition among managed care plans. These plans would be paid on the basis of a monthly fee, providing strong incentives to hold down the costs of care. Many economists favor such an approach over fee for service, which they criticize as encouraging overuse of services and failing to promote coordination of care. Further, plans competing presumably should lead to plans pushing down their premiums to attract new enrollees.

Since 1983, Medicare has offered the opportunity for its beneficiaries to enroll in managed care plans. However, unlike much of the private sector, which moved a substantial number of working families into managed care in the 1990s, Medicare has neither required such a move nor penalized those who choose to remain in fee for service. Consequently, few beneficiaries have taken advantage of these private plan options, even during the mid-1990s when such plans offered a richer benefit package than traditional Medicare. For a variety of reasons, Medicare's managed care experience has not been very positive in holding down costs to the federal government.

An active debate continues to rage, however, on whether the traditional Medicare program, or some more extensive private plan approach, will do better at restraining the growth in Medicare costs over time. What are the claims and the evidence underpinning this debate? Where should Medicare go from here? Should it provide two sets of options—fee for service and some type of managed care— with no incentives to drive beneficiaries in either direction? Or should Medicare favor private plans as implied in the recently enacted Medicare Prescription Drug Improvement and Modernization Act (MMA)? Distrust of government and reluctance of politicians to consider expanding financing for the program has pushed the debate on Medicare's future to whether the private sector can "save" Medicare.

Cost-Saving Efforts So Far

As noted in chapter 3, Medicare has a long history of attempts to slow the rate of growth of Medicare spending, mostly focused on the fee-for-service portion of the program. The introduction of an HMO option for Medicare also sought to achieve savings by paying HMOs at a rate of 95 percent of the costs for average traditional Medicare beneficiaries. So far, the fee-for-service efforts have proven to reduce Medicare spending substantially, but the evidence indicates that the opposite has been true for the managed care option. Before examining what Medicare's future should be, it is useful to consider prior successes and the sources of these savings.

Over the past 30 years, Medicare has been more successful on a per capita basis of holding down the costs of health spending growth than has private insurance. Although it is difficult to make exact comparisons, trends in the rates of growth show that Medicare and the private sector demonstrate similar patterns of growth, though on balance Medicare performed better overall than private insurance, particularly in the 1980s when Medicare was engaged in active cost savings efforts while private insurance did little in this area. During the 1990s when private insurance pushed individuals into managed care, rates of growth did come down, but not enough to catch up with the gains that Medicare made before that point. And in the late 1990s and early 2000s, Medicare once again began to widen the gap (Boccuti and Moon 2003).

What if Medicare were to be fully privatized? That would mean that all beneficiaries would need to be served by private plans, including the frailest and sickest beneficiaries. Unless good risk adjustment could be applied to compensate plans for taking such sick patients, the most vulnerable might be discouraged to enroll in a variety of ways. Traditional Medicare is currently the fallback option for a disproportionate number of the sick. If traditional Medicare were eliminated, the demand from plans for risk adjustment would likely be more intense.

Fee-for-Service Medicare

When Medicare began, a major concern of the legislation's supporters was to ensure participation by hospitals, doctors, and other providers of care. Consequently, one original principle of the program was that it not interfere with the practice of medicine. Payments were designed to be as much like standard insurance policies then in place as possible. But costs for the program rose rapidly almost from the beginning, and in the mid-1970s, it became clear that the government needed to slow spending growth. As noted in chapter 3, cost containment in fee for service was not just limited to "price controls," as critics of traditional Medicare sometimes contend. Rather, changes in Medicare have included major reforms in the structure of the payment systems that Medicare uses, affecting the volume of care as well as prices.

For example, after reforming hospital payments, Medicare now pays on the basis of the patient's diagnosis and not on what specific services are received. Since payments do not vary with a patient's length of stay in a hospital or the actual costs of the particular case, this new system encourages hospitals to be more efficient. And although the reforms initially resulted in some premature discharges, this payment system has been judged over time to be relatively successful (MedPAC 2001). Further, Medicare established peer review organizations at the same time to oversee hospitals' admission and discharge policies. Although it is difficult to judge the long-term effects of such a policy change since so many other aspects of the delivery of care have also changed, a 1991 study concluded that federal spending for Medicare hospital inpatient services declined substantially between 1981 and 1990 largely because of reductions in hospital admissions (Christensen 1991). That is, hospital spending was just 60.1 percent of what it would have been if the trend from 1975 to 1980 had continued.

Physician reforms came later and established payments on the basis of a relative value scale, initially at least limiting payments to specialists and procedures relative to more basic primary care (PPRC 1987). Many other health care insurers now use Medicare's physician relative value payment system. And in the post-acute care area, home health services are paid on the basis of an episode of care, and skilled nursing facility payments represent a bundle of specific services that used to be reimbursed separately. Most of the substantial changes in the post-acute care programs and in outpatient hospital services occurred after 1990. Nonetheless, during the 1980s, overall spending on Medicare was about 82 percent of the 1975 to 1980 trend (Christensen 1991).

After relatively little activity in the early 1990s, the 1997 Balanced Budget Act contained provisions that resulted in significantly slowing the growth in Medicare spending (discussed in more detail in chapter 3). Nearly all areas of the program were subjected to cost containment efforts with a particular emphasis on the post-acute care area (i.e., skilled nursing facility and home health benefits). As a result of these changes, spending on home health benefits actually fell in nominal dollars, reversing several years of very high rates of growth. Like both hospital and physician reforms, anticipated behavioral changes to maintain high levels of spending did not occur; rather, it seems that providers may take a considerable period of time to adapt to a new system. And although growth rates eventually began to rise over time, these mechanisms (with the exception of physician services) have had an impact on the base by holding down volume growth as well as payment levels. Legislation in the late 1990s through 2001 mitigated some of the changes, rendering the final home health payment system less restrictive than the interim system adopted right after the budget act's introduction.

All of these systems of payment require periodic updating, and analysts sometimes criticize Medicare for not adjusting quickly to new procedures. Still, the program has been a major player affecting the delivery of care. Overall, Medicare has served as a payment reform leader, fundamentally changing the way that hospitals, doctors, and other providers are paid in the United States.

The biggest question facing traditional Medicare is whether payment levels are low enough that further cost cutting will hurt access to care. If so, it becomes difficult to make further advances in cost cutting in this area. One way to assess payment levels is to compare levels of payment for Medicare with other insurers. If Medicare's payment levels fall substantially below the rates paid by others, providers may decline to treat Medicare patients. In practice, however, payment gaps have actually decreased. For example, Medicare payment amounts to physicians rose from 66 percent of private rates in 1994 to 83 percent in 2001 (Dyckman and Hess 2002), though they may have lost ground since then. Further, analyses by MedPAC (2003b) found hospital payments to be adequate and also noted that Medicare's payments relative to costs were on an upward trend while private insurers' payments came down over the 1990s. These general improvements have come about more because of the declining generosity of private payers than because of higher payment rates under Medicare. Nonetheless, Medicare has kept up in payments compared to others.

Now, however, there has been a considerable backlash from providers to private payers and to Medicare demanding higher increases in levels of allowed charges, and resulting in relatively high rates of health care spending growth from 2002 to 2004. Again, the issue of adequacy of payments and its effect on participation in Medicare needs to be closely tracked, especially for physician services. For example, payment levels for physicians were to be reduced in 2004 and 2005, but last-minute legislation prevented that. Surveys continue to show high rates of overall participation in Medicare and a willingness to accept payments without additional charges. However, in some areas of the country, evidence indicates that at least some specialists are declining to take Medicare patients (MedPAC 2004b), and some physicians threatened to pull out of Medicare unless lawmakers changed planned fee reductions in 2006.

Critics of a fee-for-service approach also criticize Medicare's administered prices as requiring elaborate price setting by government bureaucrats. How, they often ask, can we expect government workers to set prices for the thousands of physician codes and hundreds of variations in other settings? What they fail to acknowledge, however, is that private insurers use exactly the same techniques and, in fact, often use Medicare's frameworks (the hospital system based on diagnosis-related groups and the physician relative value payment scales) to set their own prices. In general, the private market for health care is not one of negotiations among equally strong buyers and sellers.

The challenge facing Medicare on service use volume is how to find ways within a fee-for-service system to encourage efficiencies beyond what has already been achieved. Medicare beneficiaries like the ability to go freely to any doctor or other provider to obtain care. There are no restrictions on visits to specialty physicians or on obtaining most diagnostic tests, for example. And it is difficult to find ways to voluntarily encourage beneficiaries to let others control their access to care. It is exactly in this area that managed care advocates point to the weakness in traditional Medicare and the potential to make such changes in private plans.

Private Plan Options

Beneficiaries have another option under the Medicare program: to enroll in a participating private plan and agree to receive their Medicare-covered services from that plan. A private plan—usually a health maintenance organization (HMO)—agrees to provide care to Medicare beneficiaries in a given area for a fixed monthly payment. Patients agree to receive care from a limited list of doctors, hospitals, and other providers. In turn, they generally face lower deductibles and coinsurance charges. When Congress established the HMO option in 1983, they intended it to save money for Medicare by paying plans at a rate of 95 percent of the costs of average enrollees. The idea was that plans would use their power to manage care to hold costs below the level of spending that occurred in fee for service, where providers face incentives to provide more care than may be necessary. Theoretically, both the government and private plans would benefit from the HMO option.

Initially, when the HMO option began, private plans attracted only a small share of Medicare beneficiaries because HMOs require beneficiaries to use only plan-approved doctors and hospitals as a condition of coverage. Medicare lagged behind the rest of the health care system in adopting managed care, in part because beneficiaries could choose to remain in fee for service with no penalties attached. To be more competitive with fee for service, many of these managed care plans offered Medicare beneficiaries such additional services as prescription drugs—a strategy that became more successful as the cost of private supplemental insurance to Medicare rose rapidly. Plans were able to offer more benefits in part because beneficiaries agreed to abide by a stricter set of rules for participation, not only by staying within a prescribed network of providers but also by obtaining permission to visit specialists or to obtain certain tests.

Plans also did well under the Medicare payment system since HMOs attracted healthier-than-average enrollees but were paid as if they were serving the average population. Not only are plans skilled at marketing to the right populations, but beneficiaries themselves are likely to sort themselves out in this way as well. Patients in the middle of a course of treatment or who rely on multiple physicians are less inclined to move into a more restricted environment and potentially disrupt their care or have to change physicians. Many studies indicate that this advantage was substantially larger than the 5 percent "discount" in payments, resulting in overpayments to private plans of at least 10 percent (GAO 2000).

With these cost advantages, plans were able to offer substantial additional benefits to those who enrolled. Lower co-payments for traditional Medicare services were common as were benefits not covered by Medicare—including drug benefits and dental and vision care, for example. In some cases, plans offered these extra benefits without an additional premium or with only a modest one. Consequently, in 1997, enrollment was booming in the HMO options and it appeared that managed care would serve a substantial share of Medicare beneficiaries. But in its 1997 annual report on the financial status of Medicare, the Board of Trustees of the Medicare trust funds indicated that costs to the government were increasing because of increasing participation in the managed care option (Board of Trustees 1997).

When the Balanced Budget Act turned to Medicare for substantial savings, bringing private plan payments in line with traditional payments became a major area for change. This legislation slowed the growth in payments to plans in recognition of the evidence that indicated that Medicare was overpaying private plans. Payments were not rolled back, but annual increases were deliberately restricted to create a "level playing field" (MedPAC 1998).

Another key area of change elicited by the Balanced Budget Act was in the breadth of private plan options. The Act established a new Part C of Medicare, called Medicare + Choice, to replace the managed care option. The intent of this change was to move Medicare farther away from its traditional role as the insurer and to expand its role as a purchaser of private insurance. Additional types of plans, such as private fee for service or physician- or hospital-led insurance, were also allowed to participate in Medicare + Choice, although only a few such alternative plans materialized. The payment slowdown overshadowed all other changes in private plans in 1997 and led to an exodus of plans from Medicare and a decline in the number of beneficiaries participating. For example, between 1999 and 2004, the share of beneficiaries with access to at least one managed care plan declined from 71 to 61 percent (MedPAC 2005).[2]

Not all withdrawals by beneficiaries occurred when plans pulled out, however. Plans that remained in the program sharply cut benefits and raised premiums. The incentives that had brought many Medicare beneficiaries into managed care were evaporating. Few beneficiaries were ever attracted to this option by the ideals of managed care, but rather for the savings they could obtain from a richer benefit package than available from traditional Medicare. In fact, many beneficiaries—even those enrolled in HMOs—indicated that they did not understand the basic principles of managed care (Kaiser Family Foundation 2000).

HMOs lobbied Congress on the unfairness of the slower payment increases compared with fee for service, omitting any acknowledgment of an overly generous base. But in some ways the HMOs were correct. The excess payments they received had enabled them to offer additional benefits and, when the payments declined, plans could not sustain the benefits needed both to attract enrollees and to effectively coordinate care. Congress modified some of the budget act changes in 1999, but HMOs remained critical of the severity of the balanced-budget cut-backs.

At the end of 2003, about 5.3 million beneficiaries participated in Medicare + Choice plans—down from a peak of more than 6.8 million in 1999 (Board of Trustees 2004). In response to the declining role of private plans, supporters of a private sector approach included further changes in the 2003 MMA. First and foremost was a substantial increase in payments—again ensuring extra plan payments above what would be necessary under the traditional fee-for-service option. In addition, the private plan option changed its name again, to Medicare Advantage. Plans are returning, but so far they are mostly plans with a history of serving Medicare. The 2003 legislation also encourages preferred provider organizations (PPOs) in the Medicare market. Many of the details still need to be worked out and it is not yet known how much expansion will come from greater PPO participation.

No one doubts that there must be change in the Medicare program in the future. Projections of greater numbers of beneficiaries and higher per capita spending ensure that either financing sources for the pro-gram must be expanded or major changes must be made in the nature of the benefits. But there has been very little serious discussion about the future. To many, the answer is dependent on a major restructuring of the program and greater reliance on private insurance. That is where most of the debate on Medicare's future has centered. Another approach—although distinctly less comprehensive—would focus on continuing to improve both private plan options and fee-for-service Medicare.

THE DEBATE OVER TRADITIONAL MEDICARE VERSUS PRIVATE PLANS

The various arguments in the debate over how best to move Medicare into the future remain both hypothetical and strongly ideological. It is important to try to sort out the various claims to understand what is at stake.

Private Plans and Competition

Claims for savings from options that shift Medicare toward a system of private insurance usually rest on two basic arguments: that the private sector is more efficient than Medicare and that competition among plans will generate more price sensitivity on the part of beneficiaries and plans alike. The federal government would subsidize a share of the costs of an average plan, leaving beneficiaries to pay the remainder. More expensive plans would require beneficiaries to pay higher premiums. The goal of such an approach is to make both plans and beneficiaries sensitive to the costs of care, leading to greater efficiency.

A particularly crucial issue on such restructuring is how the traditional Medicare program is treated. Under the current Medicare Advantage arrangement, beneficiaries are automatically enrolled in traditional Medicare unless they choose to go into a private plan. Alternatively, traditional Medicare could become just one of many (although probably more expensive) plans that beneficiaries choose from. The MMA included a proposal to create a large demonstration of such an approach beginning in 2010. Most private plan proponents prefer this approach.

Restructuring could profoundly affect Medicare's future. In particular, the traditional Medicare program could be priced beyond the means of most beneficiaries, leaving only private plan options, depending on how good the risk adjustment mechanism is and whether private plans continue to be subsidized. Further, if plans begin to sort into two groups of higher- and lower-cost plans, beneficiaries would likely be segregated into plans based on their ability to afford care. This unequal treatment would be quite different from today, where at least the basic program treats all beneficiaries alike. The details of a private sector approach will be crucial in determining both whether the government would achieve savings and the specific impacts on beneficiaries.

Advantages and Disadvantages of Private Plans

Satisfaction with managed care has generally been very high among participants, particularly if they have chosen to join from an array of possible plans. If done well, the offered coordination of care should be particularly valuable in helping to manage patients with multiple conditions or high-cost illnesses. But Medicare beneficiaries in fee for service also express considerable satisfaction with their arrangements.

Traditional Medicare and private plans face similar challenges of holding down health care spending growth. There is, in fact, no magic bullet to holding the line on such growth. Per capita spending rises because of growth in the use of services, higher prices, or a combination of the two.

On prices, Medicare's clout is well known and documented, and many private plans have found it difficult to beat Medicare on price. Indeed, in the 1990s, some of managed care's early successes relative to private indemnity plans came from the large discounts that plans with restricted networks were able to obtain. In general, Medicare payment levels were already low when private plans began to actively serve Medicare beneficiaries. The price advantage of traditional Medicare does vary by region, however, since Medicare's payments can be above or below private sector rates in specific locations.

So what about managed care's ability to control use of services? Overall, the most successful types of HMOs have always been "staff model" plans that engage in comprehensive planning and coordination of care within a tightly knit network. They are able to influence use of services and coordinate benefits. When done well, they can deliver high-quality care at lower costs than traditional indemnity programs. In practice, however, such plans are rare; the more common managed care arrangements have been loose networks of providers who join to obtain patients rather than act together in a cohesive environment of coordinated care. Studies of managed care conclude that most of them saved money by obtaining price discounts for services and not by changing the practice of health care (Lesser, Ginsburg, and Devers 2003). It is difficult to coordinate care, and many private plans have relied on arbitrary restrictions or limits that are simple to apply but that do not necessarily reflect good practice. There are too few examples of truly innovative techniques, organizational strategies, or other contributions from private plan competition. Some managed care plans, for example, do not even have the data or administrative mechanisms to attempt care coordination. Further, an insurer may see cost-effective practices where a beneficiary sees the loss of potentially essential care. Experience of managed care in the late 1990s shows that plans with stringent but arbitrary limits were largely unsuccessful and ultimately had to ease up on controls to avoid losing customers. Reining in use of services is a major future challenge for private insurance as well as for Medicare, and it is not clear which program can better curb the use of services.

PPOs are the newest type of plan suggested to improve Medicare beneficiaries' experiences. These plans are the most frequent employer-offered insurance arrangement. They are less restrictive than HMOs because individuals can see nonnetwork doctors and other care providers and still receive some reimbursement. However, PPOs generally save money by paying very little for any patient who goes outside the network for care. This strategy often shifts costs to beneficiaries. This shift may hold down PPO premiums, but from society's standpoint, it does little to help reduce overall health care costs (GAO 2004).

Another advantage of a private approach is the potential to reduce the role of government in micromanaging health care, often expressed as "no more price fixing" by government and greater flexibility for innovation and change in coverage of benefits. One of the advantages touted for private plans is their ability to be flexible and even arbitrary in making decisions. This decisionmaking ability allows private insurers to respond more quickly than a large government program can to adopt innovations and to intervene when treatments may be unnecessary. Again, however, the issue is how well this flexibility works in practice.

Society should not expect private plans to meet its goals—for example, ensuring the sickest beneficiaries receive high-quality care—if no financial incentives for the plans exist. Under the traditional Medicare program, beneficiaries do not need to fear loss of coverage when they develop health problems. This policy is vastly different from the private sector's philosophy of health coverage. Even though many private insurers are willing and able to care for Medicare patients, the easiest way to stay in business as an insurer is to seek out the healthy and avoid the sick. And in a market system with that as the dominant approach, even insurers that would like to treat sicker patients are penalized if they do so. The poor performance of the individual health insurance market in meeting the needs of persons in their early 60s and the reluctance of managed care plans under Medicare to take sick patients clearly demonstrate this problem (GAO 2000).

Private insurers want to satisfy their own customers and generate profits for stockholders. When financial incentives are very broad (such as receiving capitated—i.e., flat monthly—payments to provide all necessary care), private insurers respond as good business entities should. They seek the easiest ways of holding down the costs of providing services. This indeed is what competition is all about. Skimming of the market serves these goals very well: Medicare overpays, and plans can both satisfy the healthier beneficiaries they enroll and make good profits. These are fully legitimate responses by businesses. The problem, however, is that this response is not good for limiting overall costs to either the federal government or society as a whole. So the market should be used when we understand and approve of the direction that competition will take on health care delivery.

Finally, private insurers will almost surely have higher administrative overhead costs than does Medicare. Insurers need to advertise and promote their plans. They face a smaller risk pool that may require them to make more conservative decisions on reserves and other protections against losses over time. These plans expect to return a profit to shareholders. All of these factors cumulate and work against private companies performing better than Medicare.

Competition among Plans

Reform options that stress competition among plans seek savings not only from how private plans operate but also from competition among those plans. Often this competition includes allowing beneficiary premiums to vary: those choosing higher-cost plans pay substantially higher premiums. The theory is that beneficiaries will become more price conscious and choose lower-cost plans. This in turn will reward those private insurers able to hold down costs. Some evidence from the federal employees system and the California health insurance program for university employees suggests that this theory had disciplined the insurance market to some degree in the 1990s (Buchmueller 2000).

But the experiences in Medicare lend considerable doubt to similar cost-conscious results for the Medicare population (GAO 2000). Studies focused on retirees show much less sensitivity to price differences among older Americans. Older persons may be less willing to change doctors and learn new insurance rules just to save a few dollars each month, particularly if they have health problems and rely on several providers for the continuity of their care. Studies of retirees in California's university system, for example, indicate that while younger workers are willing to shift plans, retirees seldom change even when premiums rise dramatically (Buchmueller 2000). Experience with retirees in the Federal Employees Health Benefits program was similar when people remained in the high-option BlueCross plan despite the fact that their benefits, when coordinated with Medicare, were exactly the same as the lower-cost BlueCross option.

For a competitive model to work, at least some beneficiaries must be willing to shift plans each year (and to change providers and learn new rules) to reward the more efficient plans. Without that shift, savings for the plans will not occur. In addition, there is the question of how private insurers will respond. (If new enrollees go into such plans each year, some savings will be achieved, but these are the least costly beneficiaries and may lead to further problems as discussed below.) Will private insurers seek to improve service or instead focus on marketing and other techniques to attract a desirable, healthy patient base? It simply isn't known if the competition will really do what it is supposed to do. So undesirable outcomes may be as common as desirable ones.

In an industry like health care, where there are many examples of "market failure" (because of concentrated power, lack of good information and knowledge, product differentiation), the workings of supply and demand can lead to perverse results. For example, hospitals competing in a given area may lead to excess capacity in equipment and beds as each hospital tries to have all the latest equipment to attract doctors and patients. And as already mentioned, plans will tend to compete to attract healthy patients rather than to develop better management and care coordination protocols since the first is easier to do than the latter.

In addition, competition is emphasized as a means for moving away from a one-size-fits-all approach to insurance. Particularly as insurance becomes more expensive, why shouldn't consumers be able to choose less comprehensive plans? This approach is appropriate if that competition does not lead to risk selection or if good risk adjustment mechanisms can be applied. The difficulty is that without standardization of the most important benefits, such choice will lead to risk selection. Young, healthy 65-year-olds will pass on home health coverage, for example, in exchange for other benefits or a lower premium. But until risk adjusters improve (if ever), at least some standardization is important. Moreover, for plans to compete on price, consumers must be able to compare plans—another strong argument for at least some standardization. It is not possible to realistically expect both extensive variation in options and healthy competition.

The Implications of a Full Shift to Private Plans

Much of the opposition to a private plan approach is concern for undermining some of Medicare's strengths by moving fully to a private system or at least one in which enrollment in traditional Medicare is strongly discouraged. If private plan options remain the same as they are now, even skeptical analysts would opt for allowing access, especially to plans that demonstrate good care coordination and innovation.

Barriers for beneficiaries increase when choice becomes a necessity. For example, shifting across plans is not necessarily good for patients; it is not only disruptive, it can raise costs of care. Studies show that having one physician over a long period of time reduces costs of care (Weiss and Blustein 1996; Tang and Lansky 2005). And if only the healthier beneficiaries choose to switch plans, the sickest and most vulnerable beneficiaries may concentrate in plans that become increasingly expensive over time. The case of retirees left in the federal employees high-option BlueCross plan and a study of retirees in California suggest that even when plans become very expensive, beneficiaries may be fearful of switching and end up substantially disadvantaged (Buchmueller 2000).

Will reforms that lead to a greater reliance on the market still retain the emphasis on equal access to care and plans? For example, differential premiums could undermine some of the redistributive nature of the program that ensures even low-income beneficiaries access to high-quality care and responsive providers. Support for a market approach that moves away from "one size fits all" is a prescription for risk selection problems. About one in three Medicare beneficiaries has severe mental or physical health problems. In contrast, the healthy and relatively well off (with incomes over about $35,000 per year for singles and $45,000 for couples) make up less than 10 percent of the Medicare population. Consequently, anything that puts the sickest at greater risk relative to the healthy is out of sync with the basic tenet of Medicare. A key test of any reform should be whom it serves best.

If lawmakers eliminate the advantages of one large risk pool (such as the traditional Medicare program), they will need to find other means to ensure that insurers cannot find ways to serve only the healthy population. Although analysts have studied this very difficult challenge extensively, as yet they have not developed a satisfactory risk adjustor (Newhouse et al. 1999). Plans have, however, developed marketing tools and mechanisms to select risks. High-quality plans that attract people with extensive health care needs are likely to be more expensive than plans that focus on serving the relatively healthy. If risk adjustors are never powerful enough to level the playing field by compensating the first set of plans at a higher rate, then those with health problems, who disproportionately have lower incomes, would have to pay the highest prices under many reform schemes.

The modest gains in lower costs likely to come from increased competition and from the flexibility that the private sector enjoys could be more than offset by the loss of social insurance protection. The effort necessary to create in a private plan environment all the protections needed to compensate for moving away from traditional Medicare will be very challenging and cannot promise success. For example, even after six years (before the 2003 passage of new incentives for private plan participation), many of the provisions in the 1997 Balanced Budget Act that would be essential in any further moves to emphasize private insurance—generating new ways of paying private plans, improving risk adjustment, and developing information for beneficiaries—were not fully put in place before the latest round of legislation intended to promote private plans.

Finally, it is not clear that there is a full appreciation by policymakers or the public at large of all the consequences of a competitive market. Potential advantages of relying on private plans for serving the Medicare population include choice among competing plans and the discipline that such competition can bring to prices and innovation. But if there is to be choice and competition, some plans will not do well in a particular market and, as a result, they will leave. In fact, if no plans ever left, that would likely be a sign that competition was not working well. But plan withdrawals will result in disruptions and complaints by beneficiaries—much like those that occurred with the withdrawals from Medicare+Choice. Beneficiaries must then find another private plan or return to traditional Medicare. They may have to choose new doctors and learn new rules. This situation has led to politically charged discussions about payment levels in the program even though that is only one of many factors that may cause plans to withdraw. Thus, not only will beneficiaries be unhappy, but there may be strong political pressure to keep federal payments higher than a well-functioning market would require.

BALANCING THE PRIVATE MARKET AND TRADITIONAL MEDICARE APPROACHES

Another strategy is to improve both traditional Medicare and private plan options. Although purists on both sides of the debate may not be satisfied with a middle-ground compromise, uncertainties around a full move to private plans may warrant it. Beneficiaries' choices when faced with both options could help decide the future of Medicare. Further, it makes little sense to look for a solution that takes policymakers permanently out of Medicare's future. The flux and complexity of our health care system will necessitate continuing attention to this program.

Private plans can play an important role and may innovate on their own. But in much the same way that we view basic research on medicine as requiring a public component, innovations in health delivery also need such support. These innovations in treatment and coordination of care should focus on those with substantial health problems— exactly the population that many private plans seek to avoid. Some private plans might be willing to specialize in individuals with specific needs, but that is not going to happen in an environment emphasizing price competition and with barely adequate risk adjustors. Reform needs to focus on enhancing the effectiveness of private plans by rewarding such innovation. Further, the default plan should be traditional Medicare for those who cannot choose. So there needs to be a strong commitment to maintaining a traditional Medicare program while seeking to define the appropriate role for alternative options.

Providing additional flexibility to the Centers for Medicare and Medicaid Services (CMS) to manage and develop payment initiatives aimed at using competition where appropriate also could result in long-term cost savings that serve patients well. In the areas of durable medical equipment and perhaps even some testing and laboratory services, contracting could be used to obtain favorable prices. The 2003 legislation allows CMS to establish demonstrations to improve fee for service—that is, by seeking changes that do not go as far as full capitation and managed care. Giving doctors incentives to coordinate and manage care for their patients through a less rigorously controlled system would likely be attractive to many patients, especially if they are convinced that solid medical evidence backs up the coordination efforts. These are but a few of the options that ought to be considered.

In addition, better norms and standards of care could provide quality of care protections to all Americans. Investment in outcomes research, disease management, and other techniques to improve patient treatment will require a substantial public commitment. The investment of time and resources cannot be done as well in a proprietary, for-profit environment where dissemination of new ways of coordinating care may not be shared.

Critics of Medicare rightly point out that the inadequacy of its benefit package has resulted in an inefficient system that forces most beneficiaries to rely on two sources of insurance to meet their needs. Some argue that improvements in coverage can only occur in combination with structural reform. Some advocates of a private approach to insurance go further, suggesting that the structural reform itself will naturally produce benefit improvements. This argument implicitly holds the debate on improved benefits hostage to accepting other unrelated changes. That logic actually should run in the other direction. It is not reasonable to expect any number of other changes to work without first offering a more comprehensive benefit package for Medicare. The fee-for-service system could be changed in ways that might encourage better care delivery if the benefit package were to be restructured. Restructuring would also allow payments made to private plans to improve, allowing them to better coordinate care. For example, it is not reasonable to ask patients to participate in a program to reduce hypertension (which can save costs over the long run) without covering the prescription drugs that are likely to be an essential part of that effort. In addition, a better benefit package will also allow at least some beneficiaries to forego the purchase of inefficient private supplemental insurance. That alone should be a goal of reform and is the subject of the next chapter.

6

HOW COULD THE BENEFIT STRUCTURE BE IMPROVED?

M edicare's critics often refer to Medicare as an anachronism, a 1965 Cadillac on today's superhighways. This is certainly the case for the structure and composition of Medicare's basic benefit package. Parts of the program look very much like private insurance did in 1965. Medicare's specific cost-sharing pieces were established ad hoc from political horse-trading and concerns about limiting the program's costs. The benefit package did not expand substantially until 2003,[1] despite general agreement since the 1970s that the benefit structure should change to reflect new beneficiary needs and evolving private insurance. And even in 2003, the only improvements in benefits under traditional Medicare were the addition of a stand-alone drug plan and several new preventive benefits.

The lack of progress on improving benefits is partly due to a major conflict over whether changes should only come in the context of broader reforms. That was the trade-off required for adding a prescription drug benefit to Medicare in 2003. Regardless of other changes in Medicare, an improved benefit package beyond the new drug benefit is needed for *either* traditional Medicare or private plans to work well. The 2003 legislation implicitly recognized the need to expand benefits further by requiring the new preferred provider organizations promoted in the law to have stop-loss protections and a combined deductible for Parts A and B (see the discussion in chapter 1 and appendix A for more information about Medicare's structure). But it did not make similar changes to traditional Medicare, which will remain the dominant source of care for the foreseeable future.

Deciding Where to Start

Creating a more comprehensive benefit package for Medicare requires consideration of several key issues. First, the inadequacy of the current benefit package puts an inordinate burden on most Medicare beneficiaries. Particularly for the elderly, those with low incomes, and those with high health care needs, the costs resulting from excluded services and high cost sharing lead to substantial out-of-pocket spending. Such expenses often force people to choose between health care and other vital goods and services, or even among various health care needs.

Those who can afford it turn to private supplemental insurance to fill the coverage gaps. But individual Medigap plans do not, on balance, reduce overall costs, though they do make health coverage for seniors more complex. As noted in chapter 1, both employer retiree coverage and Medicaid add good protections, but employer coverage is shrinking and states are struggling to keep up their Medicaid programs.

Medicare's high cost-sharing requirements vary between Part A (Hospital Insurance) and Part B (Supplementary Medical Insurance), resulting in complicated rules treating different services differently. Further, there is no upper bound on the amount of cost sharing that can be assessed. Such upper-bound protections are referred to as "stop-loss." Over time, Part A cost sharing, which is linked to increases in the costs of hospital payments, has become very expensive. But the Part A deductible, set at $952 in 2005, does little in practice to discourage unnecessary use of services since the decision to enter a hospital is not up to the individual. And those unlucky enough to trigger the hospital coinsurance face thousands of dollars in cost-sharing liability. The Part B deductible, however, is quite low at $124 per year. But those with very high expenses pay at least 20 percent of the cost of most Part B services with no upper payment limit. As a consequence, Part B cost sharing is the main expense for those in the top 20 percent of Medicare cost sharing. Figure 6.1 shows a breakdown of the basic Medicare liability created for an average beneficiary and for one in the top fifth of Medicare spending, indicating that Part B co-payments account for two-thirds of Medicare's overall cost sharing and only a little less than that for those in the top fifth.

But this Medicare liability, which is the amount that Medicare requires of beneficiaries (or someone paying on their behalf), does not

Figure 6.1. Source of Medicare Liability, 2004

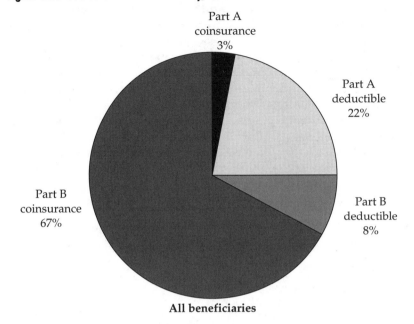

All beneficiaries

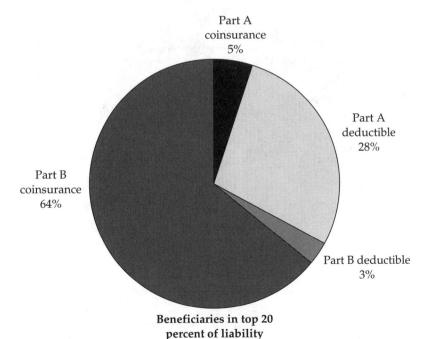

**Beneficiaries in top 20
percent of liability**

Source: American Institutes for Research calculations from 2001 Medicare Current Beneficiaries Survey (MCBS).

tell the full story of what happens to beneficiaries. When individuals purchase private supplemental insurance or receive it gratis from former employers or Medicaid, they are shielded from some of the direct cost-sharing amounts. However, cost sharing still affects these beneficiaries since most of them pay part or all of the supplemental premium costs, and any increase in cost sharing is likely to be passed on directly through higher supplemental premiums. The overall generosity of the benefit package also affects those in HMOs, since the benefit package determines the average contribution the government makes to the HMO. If that contribution falls (because of a cost-sharing increase in traditional Medicare, for example), the HMO beneficiary's premiums will likely increase.

Figure 6.2 indicates the various components of spending that beneficiaries undertake toward the cost of the care. Note that prescription

Figure 6.2 Distribution of Out-of-Pocket Spending Among Elderly Beneficiaries, 2004

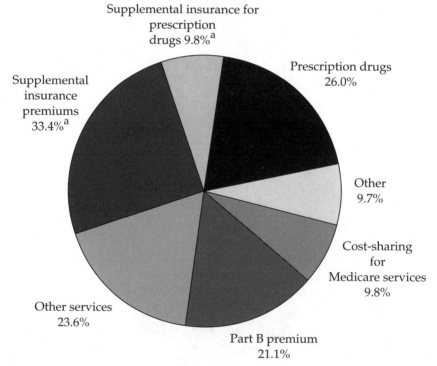

Supplemental insurance for prescription drugs 9.8%[a]

Prescription drugs 26.0%

Supplemental insurance premiums 33.4%[a]

Other 9.7%

Cost-sharing for Medicare services 9.8%

Other services 23.6%

Part B premium 21.1%

Source: American Institutes for Research Analysis of the 2000 Medicare Current Beneficiary Survey, projected to 2004.

[a] Together, insurance accounts for 43.2 percent of beneficiary spending. The portion attributed to drugs is pulled out here.

drugs account for a little more than a third of the out-of-pocket costs of older Americans. High out-of-pocket spending on drugs has received most of the attention in recent years. These burdens will ease in 2006 for those who enroll in the new drug plans. For example, if the level of protection that will be available in 2006 had been offered in 2004, the out-of-pocket spending by Medicare beneficiaries in traditional Medicare would fall from an average of $3,368 to $2,922. So prescription drug coverage will only modestly lower the overall costs. Beneficiaries are still likely to be concerned about Medicare's other cost-sharing liabilities, especially the lack of stop-loss protections. Improvements in these areas would help all beneficiaries who either pay the costs directly or are responsible for paying for at least part of their supplemental insurance costs.

For example, lowering the hospital deductible would benefit both those hospitalized and anyone who purchases supplemental insurance since the actuarial cost of providing that gap-filling insurance and hence the premium should fall. The existence of supplemental coverage that pays for the cost sharing makes it difficult to ensure that cost sharing will have its intended effect. Further, it is difficult to determine exactly who benefits when changes are made in cost-sharing liability because supplemental insurance can blunt the redistributional impact of any changes by spreading the costs of any changes over the whole group of insureds as opposed to those using the services.

Not all of the redistributional impact is necessarily eliminated for those with supplemental insurance, however. Some sensitivity to where cost-sharing changes are made arises in Medigap (the private insurance purchased directly by individuals) because most Medigap premiums have become age-rated, meaning that older persons pay much more on average than do those ages 65 to 69. These differences can vary by as much as a factor of 2 or 3 to 1. So to the extent that changes in cost sharing ease liabilities for the very old—who happen to disproportionately use services such as hospitals and post-acute care—the types of changes discussed here would be of at least indirect benefit in reducing burdens on many of the sickest beneficiaries who rely on Medigap or who have no supplemental coverage.

Together, those who rely on Medicare or on Medicare and Medigap represent about 4 out of every 10 beneficiaries. And they are disproportionately concentrated in the group earning between 150 percent and 250 percent of the federal poverty level (FPL). These are the beneficiaries for whom the *specifics* of cost-sharing changes make the most difference.

Particularly in the case of Medigap coverage, the cost of the insurance is greater, on average, than the benefits provided since individuals pay both the actuarial costs of the benefits plus administrative costs and profits of the insurers. In any given year, Medigap can prevent individuals from facing very high expenses. But over time, Medigap is not a very good deal for beneficiaries because its administrative costs are very high. Further, across the standard plans offered, there tends to be considerable risk selection as people with high expenses choose the more comprehensive Medigap options (especially those with some drug coverage) (Alexcih et al. 1997). Consequently, the actuarial costs for those plans are very high. And for the very old, who have to pay high premiums because of the pricing structure that most insurers use, the costs can reach $3,000 to $4,000 annually.

MAJOR CHANGES IN THE BENEFIT STRUCTURE

Improving benefits by enough so that supplemental coverage is not necessary would have a major impact on Medicare. If that happens, not only would the cost sharing be distributed as intended, but additional savings to beneficiaries would arise by alleviating the costs and complications of having two insurance policies. Persons with Medigap, Medicare only, and those in Medicare Advantage would all benefit from improvements, even if they pay increased premiums for such coverage. And as employers shift more of the costs onto their retirees through higher premiums and other changes, an expanded benefit package could help those beneficiaries by slowing the trend to reduce employer benefits or by filling in the gaps for those who lose coverage.

Ideally, an expanded benefit package for Medicare beneficiaries would create insurance comparable to that held by many younger families, with a prescription drug benefit and improved cost-sharing structure. The drug benefit just beginning in 2006 will cover less than what many younger workers have, however, and as mentioned above, other cost sharing remains unchanged. To achieve a more comprehensive structure, benefits would need to be expanded on both fronts.

In a benefit package modeled after the BlueCross BlueShield plan for federal employees, the amount Medicare covers (based on 2004 costs) would raise the actuarial value of Medicare from $5,435 (with no drug benefits) to $7,251 under a "Medicare Extra" benefit (Davis et al. 2005).[2] This benefit package would differ from traditional Medicare by limiting cost sharing to a combined deductible of $250, a stop-loss of $2,000, Part B coinsurance of 10 percent, and a drug benefit with a 25 percent co-payment.

The premium that beneficiaries pay could be increased—by about $90 per month—to keep such an option budget neutral. But with the burden of the other premiums (for Parts B and D), the cost would likely be beyond the reach of many low- and modest-income families not eligible for Medicaid. Further, policymakers are often very reluctant to generate higher premiums because they are such a visible part of the Medicare program. The advantage of providing greater protections for those with high expenses is often forgotten in the furor over higher premiums. The insurance value of benefits is often ignored in the rush to calculate winners and losers of any policy change. This was one of the major lessons of the repealed 1988 Medicare Catastrophic Coverage Act (see chapter 4).

A rough sense of the overall costs of this proposal (if the government absorbed the costs) can be obtained by multiplying the per capita averages by 42 million, the number of beneficiaries on the program in 2004. On a base of $312 billion in spending in 2004, Medicare spending as a result of this expansion would rise by about $45 billion if applied to all beneficiaries. Since a substantial number of Medicare beneficiaries are currently eligible for both Medicare and Medicaid, there would be some offsetting cost reductions for both state and federal governments.

Alternatively, the expansion could be treated as a Medicare option, allowing people to choose between the limited traditional package and "Medicare Extra." In this case, individuals would pay the differential premium themselves, likely in lieu of Medigap. Medicare Extra might face adverse selection, however, if, as a voluntary option, its premiums rise by more than an additional $90 per month.

This option could also be done in concert with an increase in financial protections for those with low or modest incomes, since such individuals now find it hard to purchase private insurance and would be sensitive to mandatory premium increases. Sliding-scale premiums could both protect those with the lowest incomes and expand the income-related premium from the Medicare Prescription Drug Improvement and Modernization Act of 2003.

LESS COMPREHENSIVE APPROACHES

A more modest, but still positive, impact on beneficiaries could be achieved even if beneficiaries still take out supplemental policies. First, the simple creation of expanded coverage under Medicare would better spread the risks of health care since Medicare's premium is community-rated (i.e., it does not rise with age). And if the protections are particularly concentrated on those with high risks, risk selection issues affecting the purchase of Medigap could be somewhat mitigated as discussed earlier. Finally, if Medigap's high administrative costs discouraged beneficiaries from purchasing it, many would be better off. Costs would likely fall to the government if beneficiaries faced modest cost sharing.[3] In a climate reluctant to expand government, this approach may be the most to expect, particularly for the basic Medicare-covered services.

Criteria for Assessing Changes in the Benefit Package

To realize the greatest impact from a modest set of changes in cost sharing, a number of factors ought to be considered, including

- reducing costs for high users of Medicare services and persons with chronic conditions and
- recognizing the need for some balance between benefits for high users and other beneficiaries to ensure that the benefits are not limited to catastrophic protection.

These are competing factors that must be weighed in considering various options. For example, stop-loss protections set at high levels will help high users of services but do little for the vast majority of Medicare beneficiaries. And combined with an increase in the Part B premium to help offset the costs of a stop-loss improvement, the majority of beneficiaries will face higher, not lower, costs. Alternatively, those with chronic conditions might have substantial out-of-pocket spending on drugs, but less on hospital and other Medicare-covered services. In that case, beneficiaries might prefer improvements in the drug benefit over other changes. As people age, their cost-sharing liability increases. Persons age 85 and older, for example, have cost sharing averaging 86 percent higher than those ages 65 to 74.

Tables 6.1–6.3 show several measures that aid in the evaluation of various options. The first column shows the per capita change in Medicare liability, which is the average across all beneficiaries and indicates the relative costs of a particular option. Options that display the same average change would generate about equal costs or savings to the federal government. The second column is the average change for the 20 percent of beneficiaries who face the highest Medicare liability. These are the "high users" of services. The third and fourth columns show the percentage of beneficiaries experiencing a decrease or an increase in liability, allowing an examination of how significant the change might appear to various individuals. As many would face cost-sharing increases, it may be difficult to convince beneficiaries that this is indeed a benefit improvement. Proposals to alter Medicare's cost-sharing structure often include three changes: rebalancing the deductibles for Parts A and B, adding stop-loss protections, and adding co-pays for laboratory services and home health benefits.

Medicare's Deductibles

Much of the criticism directed at Medicare's cost sharing in recent years has focused on the two deductibles. Part A's deductible is much larger than Part B's—$952 vs. $124 in 2006. Initially, the Part B deductible was larger ($50 vs. $40 for Part A), but the Part A deductible was tied to the cost of hospitalization and thus grew rapidly. Part B has increased only sporadically. Ironically, insurers often recognize that physician services are subject to more discretion than hospital care and establish a higher deductible for physician services than for hospital services. Proposals to change cost sharing either change the value of each or combine the two deductibles.[4]

In practice, the two approaches have quite different redistributional impacts. For example, the first pair of options in table 6.1 contrasts a combined $600 deductible with an increase in the B deductible to $200 (and no change in the Part A deductible). These changes would save costs to the federal government by about $67 per beneficiary. In this case, savings to those in the highest quintile would be about $662 with the combined deductible, while cost sharing would rise in that quintile if the only change is an increase in the B deductible. Nearly 20 percent of beneficiaries would have a decrease in their overall liabilities under the combined deductible option. Yet for those with modest expenses, costs would rise by a greater amount than under the Part B deductible–only change.

Second, consider an example that would only modestly increase average beneficiary liability. If the Part A deductible were reduced to $500 and assessed no more than once in any given year, while the Part B deductible rose to $350 annually, average per capita cost sharing

Table 6.1. Impacts of Possible Changes in Medicare Deductibles

Option	Average change in cost sharing ($)	Average change in cost sharing for top quintile of liability ($)	Percent with cost sharing decrease	Percent with cost sharing increase
A/B combined deductible of $600	+ 67	− 662	19	67
B deductible of $200	+ 68	+ 80	0	86
A/B combined deductible of $500	+ 9	− 742	19	67
B deductible of $350 and A deductible of $500 (once per year)	+ 12	− 487	19	67

Source: American Institutes for Research calculations based on 2001 Medicare Current Beneficiary Survey, projected to 2004.

would rise by about $12. A nearly equivalent increase in liability of $9 would arise from a combined A/B deductible of $500. Beneficiaries in the top quintile of Medicare liability again would be better off with a combined deductible even though the hospital deductible is reduced in the first option of this pair. That is, the reduction in cost sharing for those in the top 20 percent of Medicare cost sharing would be about $255 more than for the two separate deductibles. The shares of people affected by either an increase or decrease are the same.

Stop-Loss Protection

One of the areas of greatest concern to health policy professionals assessing the quality of health insurance is whether it offers good stop-loss protection—that is, the guarantee that above a certain threshold, the individual should not have to continue to pay out of pocket for covered services. One of Medicare's greatest weaknesses is the lack of an upper limit on the amount of cost sharing that beneficiaries are theoretically liable to pay.

Most private plans offer stop-loss protection, but Medicare has no such provision. Beneficiaries with complicated illnesses (and no supplemental insurance) can end up owing tens of thousands of dollars toward the costs of Medicare-covered services. This is particularly the case under Part B of the program, where the 20 percent coinsurance can become quite large for those with extensive medical bills. Part B cost sharing constitutes about 75 percent of all Medicare cost-sharing liabilities (figure 6.1).

Ironically, many beneficiaries do not see the lack of stop-loss protection as the coverage problem. Traditionally, Medicare enrollees have been more concerned about choosing supplemental policies on the basis of first-dollar rather than last-dollar coverage. Further, objections to the Medicare catastrophic legislation in 1988 were that the benefits were not the ones enrollees most desired or valued. Nonetheless, adding good stop-loss protection to Medicare would be an important improvement in the program's fundamental insurance function.

The higher the stop-loss cutoff, the less expensive the protection. But the disparity in incomes across beneficiaries always creates a dilemma. For example, a $5,000 cutoff is low enough to be expensive to add to Medicare but high enough to represent a substantial share of income for modest-income families to pay before hitting the stop-loss limit. To be budget neutral would require an increase of nearly $10 per month in premiums, though only a very small share of beneficiaries would reach that stop-loss threshold in any year.

Table 6.2 indicates a number of stop-loss-only benefit options. Even when the stop-loss is $4,000 at an average cost to the government of

Table 6.2. Impacts of Possible Stop-Loss Options

Stop-loss amount ($)	Average change in cost sharing ($)	Change in cost sharing for top quintile of liability ($)	Percent with cost sharing increase
2,000	−366	−1,833	16
3,000	−241	−1,206	10
4,000	−163	−817	6
5,000	−116	−578	4

Source: American Institutes for Research calculations based on 2001 Medicare Current Beneficiary Survey, projected to 2004.

$163 per beneficiary, its impact on the top quintile generates an average reduction in spending of $817 and lower cost sharing for just 6 percent of beneficiaries. Costs rise steadily as the upper limit is lowered. If the only change made is to add stop-loss protection, the upper limit that would be relatively inexpensive may turn out to be so high that few people would view this as substantial protection.

Combining Stop-Loss and Deductible Changes

What happens when deductible changes are combined with the addition of a stop-loss? Does the combined deductible still appear to be a more favorable approach? Also, are combinations better than using a stop-loss-only approach? Table 6.3 illustrates options that combine stop-loss with other changes. In the first set of examples, the overall costs to the government are in the range of $120 per beneficiary—either a $4.9 billion increase in government liabilities or a $10 added Medicare premium (depending on whether the change increases government costs or is shifted to beneficiaries).

Again, the results show that a combined deductible produces generally better results for the high users of services and for spreading reductions in cost sharing across a broader share of beneficiaries. At the level of spending being discussed, a stop-loss-only option must be set at $5,000, limiting the share of beneficiaries who benefit to 4 percent. The option that keeps separate A and B deductibles and raises the B deductible to $350 generates enough to lower the stop-loss to $3,000. This change expands the share of the population facing lower cost sharing. But for the share of individuals helped and the size of the benefit to those in the top 20 percent of Medicare liability, the combined deductible does considerably better. That is, although the stop-loss is $4,000, a number of people who would have faced higher Part A deductibles but who might not reach a stop-loss of $3,000 are also helped. Essentially, such an approach offers two types of benefits for

Table 6.3. Impacts of Possible Combinations of Cost Sharing Changes, 2004

Option	Average change in cost sharing ($)	Average change in cost sharing for top quintile of liability ($)	Percent with cost sharing decrease	Percent with cost sharing increase
Stop-loss of $5,000	−116	−578	4	0
A/B combined deductible of $450, stop-loss of $4,000	−124	−1,301	20	67
B deductible of $350, A deductible of $876, and stop-loss of $3,000	−113	−1,180	11	75
Stop-loss of $3,000	−241	−1,206	10	0
A/B combined deductible of $500, stop-loss of $2,000	−236	−1,968	22	64
B deductible of $350, A deductible of $876, and stop-loss of $2,000	−241	−1,819	16	70

Source: American Institutes for Research calculations using the 2001 Medicare Current Beneficiary Survey, projected to 2004.

Note: A and B refer to the two major parts of the Medicare program. When there is a separate A deductible, it applies no more than once per year, unlike current law.

persons who are hospitalized: the lower hospital deductible reduces the likelihood of going above the stop-loss limit, but it is also there as a protection for those with very high expenses from Part B (i.e., physician and other services for a hospital stay).

The second set of options, which would be about twice as expensive to offer, again demonstrates that it is better to change the deductibles to obtain a lower stop-loss when the goal is to provide better catastrophic protection. And the combined deductible continues to help a larger share of beneficiaries by a greater amount than when only the Part B deductible increases.[5]

Finally, although a $3,000 stop-loss is not exceptionally generous—particularly since it does not include prescription drug costs—it may be sufficient to allow some beneficiaries to forego the purchase of Medigap to save even more. As private insurance has become less comprehensive, modest improvements in Medicare's basic package (along with prescription drug coverage) may begin to look more and more like coverage in the private sector.

The difficulty with all these approaches, however, is that while rearranging cost sharing improves insurance protections against large losses, many individual beneficiaries would face higher cost sharing in any given year. Policymakers have been reluctant to make such changes in the past. But they have been equally unwilling to soften the blow by having the federal government absorb some of the additional costs of improving catastrophic protection. The dilemma of the 1988 catastrophic legislation continues.

Other Cost-Sharing Changes

A favorite proposal by many who would like to see cost sharing expanded to all Medicare services is to apply it to home health services and/or laboratory services, since these two areas currently have no cost-sharing requirements. Before the Balanced Budget Act of 1997, home health spending was rising rapidly and many critics cited lack of cost sharing as a contributor. But the legislative changes to shift home health payments to a prospective system led first to a drop in the use of home health services and then to much slower growth in those services over time. In fact, the advent of a prospective payment system has many analysts worried about too few services being provided rather than too many. Nonetheless, adding home health cost sharing remains a favorite suggestion of those seeking Medicare cuts.

A major problem with adding cost sharing to home health is that a small number of very frail beneficiaries uses home health care services. Such beneficiaries are likely to be already subject to high cost sharing as heavy users of other health care services. A stop-loss could reduce the negative impact of a home health co-pay, but it would still result in high cost sharing for the most vulnerable members of the population.

The latest round of budget options that the Congressional Budget Office presents each year (CBO 2005) includes an estimate of the savings from imposing a 10 percent co-payment on the total costs of each home health episode. An estimated savings of $2.3 billion would occur if fully implemented in 2007. Although no detailed simulation results are presented here, it is important to note that the very old and those with disabilities would be disproportionately disadvantaged. Their costs would be higher than the average by a factor of about 4 to 1, increasing the costs on the most vulnerable and persons with chronic conditions.

The same is likely to be the case for increased cost sharing on laboratory expenses. Because beneficiaries have little control over the tests they receive, legislators dropped cost sharing on laboratory services in 1984. In this case, cost sharing is likely to do little to change laboratory services use. Moreover, this policy change simplified payments to labs because they do not have to bill patients directly. CBO (2005) estimated $1.2 billion in savings from a 20 percent co-pay in 2007—savings of less than one-half of 1 percent of overall spending on the program in that year.

Overall, the cost-sharing requirements in Medicare need to examine whether these payments are being used merely to lower costs by passing higher burdens to beneficiaries or whether they truly help to moderate health care spending. If the latter is a goal, then changes in cost sharing need to be carefully targeted and reduced in areas where behavior is unlikely to change because of the imposition or expansion of cost-sharing requirements.

CHANGING THE NEW PRESCRIPTION DRUG BENEFIT

As described in chapter 4, the benefit available to beneficiaries in 2006 contains a major gap in coverage—the so-called "doughnut hole." Beneficiaries have coverage for expenses above and below that gap. Why did this legislation create such a complicated benefit structure? Foremost, the framers were attempting to limit spending on the new drug benefit. And because the goals were to provide both some catastrophic protection and encourage participation (since the plans are usually voluntary) of those with low expenses, the only way to do so was to create a gap in the middle. Ironically, this gap is exactly where expenses are rising most rapidly and for those drugs that have the potential to save costs over time. It would be expensive to fill the gap because the hole affects more than 40 percent of beneficiaries (see chapter 4). There are, however, several options for eliminating the gap. Filling in the gap with 75 percent coverage—that is, simply extending the coverage that will be available for the $251–$2,250 range spent to the $2,251–$5,100 range as well—would increase federal costs by about 43 percent above the basic amount in 2006.

Just as is the case with changing coverage in Parts A and B, a comprehensive change is unlikely. However, other options that would reduce coverage below $2,250 in spending to help finance the gap's elimination would raise federal liabilities by smaller amounts, as shown in table 6.4. In fact, reducing the coverage by raising the deductible and increasing the coinsurance for spending below $2,250 would allow half of all spending on drugs to be covered up to $5,100. This option is likely the most straightforward, but other combinations, some requiring a modest premium increase, could also be implemented. Although there is some risk of healthier beneficiaries not signing up, the current penalties for delaying are very strong.

Table 6.4. Costs of Filling in the Drug Benefit "Doughnut Hole"

Option	Costs as share of existing benefit (%)
Baseline: $250 deductible, 25% co-pay $251–$2,250, 100% co-pay $2,251–$5,100, 5% co-pay above $5,100	100
Option 1: $250 deductible, 25% co-pay $251–$5,100, 5% co-pay above $5,100	143
Option 2: $400 deductible, 50% co-pay $401–$5,100, 5% co-pay above $5,100	105
Option 3: $250 deductible, 50% co-pay $251–$5,000, 5% co-pay above $5,000	119

Source: American Institutes for Research calculations using the 2001 Medicare Current Beneficiary Survey, projected to 2004.

Research indicates that focusing solely on the new prescription drug benefit may not be the appropriate next step for improving coverage. While eliminating the coverage gap makes considerable sense for simplifying benefits under Medicare, it does not do as well in protecting the most vulnerable against high out-of-pocket liabilities. Instead, changing the structure of inpatient and outpatient cost sharing can provide better protection for vulnerable beneficiaries. The impact of such changes is more directly concentrated among those with high Medicare liabilities. Additional funding to eliminate the doughnut hole is not as effective as budget-neutral improvements to Parts A and B for helping beneficiaries with high medical expenses, poor health status, and cognitive and physical disabilities (Angeles and Moon forthcoming).

THE SPECIAL CASE OF PERSONS WITH LOW INCOMES

This chapter has focused on the overall benefit package offered under Medicare and has not considered the special issues of those with low incomes. A $3,000 stop-loss, for example, is well above "catastrophe" for many with low incomes. This issue needs to be considered separately and becomes complicated when determining whether Medicare or Medicaid should be responsible. Considering special treatment for those with low incomes raises issues of equity across geographic areas, the level of responsibility left to the states, and whether the perception of Medicare beneficiaries with low incomes will be as mainly participating in the welfare-based Medicaid program. Other issues include how to determine eligibility (e.g., whether an asset test will be used), how any phaseout of benefits would occur, and what, if any, cost sharing is appropriate for beneficiaries higher up the income scale.

In addition, the specific income cutoff level not only affects the number of low-income persons given special protections, but also makes changes in the basic benefit package for those with higher incomes more palatable. That is, the higher the income cutoff for low-income protections, the less generous the basic benefit package may need to be. For example, stop-loss protection of $4,000 will not be helpful for singles with incomes of $15,000 since that would mean they would have to devote 27 percent of their incomes just for Medicare cost sharing. More generous stop loss protections for those with low-incomes up to 150 or 200 percent of the poverty level could make a $4,000 stop-loss a more justifiable cutoff for those to whom it would apply. A lower-level stop loss could then be set for beneficiaries whose incomes are below 150 percent of FPL (as it is under the new drug benefit). At 150 percent of FPL, protections extend to singles with incomes of $14,280 or less and couples with incomes of $17,321 or less in 2005. For these beneficiaries, the cutoff might be set at $1,500 or $2,000. But as the income cutoff level increases, so do the number of people affected and the cost of enhanced protections, as shown in table 6.5. If the protections extended to as high as 200 percent of FPL, nearly half of Medicare beneficiaries would be eligible, greatly increasing the cost of offering such protections. In choosing some combination, the lower the income cutoff, the lower the stop loss should be. If there were also an asset test, the proportion eligible would likely fall substantially since asset limits tend to be quite stringent (Moon, Friedland, and Shirey 2002). For example, the Congressional Budget Office estimated that the asset tests under the new drug benefit would reduce protections for about 1.8 million of the 6.4 million beneficiaries who would qualify for protec-

Table 6.5. Cost Increases to Stop Loss Proposal if Lower Limit Is Provided to Beneficiaries with Low Incomes

Stop loss cutoff for low-income beneficiaries ($)	Increase in costs if offered to persons below (percent)		
	100% of FPL	150% of FPL	200% of FPL
1,000	68	97	132
1,500	37	68	91
2,000	25	46	63
2,500	17	31	42

Source: American Institutes for Research Calculations from MCBS.

Note: Assumes stop loss of $4,000 for those above the federal poverty level (FPL) cutoffs. FPL = federal poverty level.

tions on the basis of income (CBO 2004). The share of beneficiaries affected by an asset test also rises as income cutoffs go up.

Finally, given the large number of Medicare beneficiaries with modest incomes, the cost of improving the drug benefit just to low-income persons could be quite high, particularly if that protection is comprehensive. For example, the Congressional Budget Office (2004) estimated that these protections constituted about one-half of the costs of the prescription drug benefit when they extend only up to 135 percent of FPL for full benefits and 150 percent of FPL for partial protection.

Conclusions

Adding a prescription drug benefit to Medicare was a timely and important change in the program. It is, however, insufficient to eliminate the need for supplemental insurance. Indeed, since the drug benefit is a stand-alone option for those in traditional Medicare, most people will end up with three types of insurance: basic Medicare, a drug policy, and a supplemental policy to fill in other coverage gaps— not a desirable outcome for most beneficiaries. The need for multiple insurance policies will exacerbate the complexity of health insurance for seniors and persons with disabilities. A better approach would be to expand basic benefits to allow most beneficiaries to forego the purchase of Medigap. If improving protections for high-cost beneficiaries is the goal, adding stop-loss protections for traditional Medicare-covered services is the logical next step to expand benefits. And as indicated in this chapter, some of the changes that could achieve this end are not inordinately expensive if combined with other changes in the structure of Medicare's deductibles. Further, because of the large number of Medicare beneficiaries with incomes just above the poverty level, offering enhanced protections up the income scale will be difficult to accomplish because of its high costs.

7

WHO SHOULD PAY?

One crucial, but often ignored, aspect of Medicare's future is who should pay for the program. In a political environment of "no new taxes," few policymakers are willing to increase resources to the program. But implicitly, this means that the beneficiaries (or their families) must pay. Proposals to find additional ways to reduce the costs of providing health care to disabled and elderly Americans that eliminate unnecessary care or achieve greater efficiencies can reduce the overall bill for the program. But options for "saving money" under Medicare that simply shift costs onto beneficiaries implicitly answer the question of who should pay with "beneficiaries, not taxpayers."

Yet the choices are seldom expressed that directly. Rather, in response to questions about the sustainability of Medicare, the usual answers tend to be that beneficiaries must bear a greater share of the costs, or that age of eligibility must change. But this sidesteps the question of who *should* pay by indicating that while we as a society cannot afford the taxes to pay for health care for an aging population, the elderly and disabled themselves can somehow afford to do so.

As indicated in chapter 2, the combined effect of rising health care costs and an aging population (a growing share of the total population) will hike Medicare spending as a share of gross domestic product (GDP). Medicare trustees project that Medicare spending will rise from its current share of about 2.7 percent of GDP to nearly 6.8 percent in 2030 (Boards of Trustees 2005). The new prescription drug benefit is one cost escalator that ensures the Medicare program will cover a greater *share* of health care spending for beneficiaries than at present.

But it is also important to note that the 6.8 percent figure includes premiums and taxes paid by Medicare beneficiaries themselves. So the burden on taxpayers (who are not also beneficiaries) is smaller—less than 6 percent of GDP. Also, over this period, the share of income spent by seniors and persons with disabilities will rise due to the same health care cost increases that help drive up Medicare's spending. If, as discussed earlier, beneficiaries (and their families) continue to pay the same share of total acute care costs as at present (after adjusting for the new drug benefit), they will effectively pay an amount equivalent to about 2.5 percent of GDP in 2030.[1] The appropriate question for Medicare is how to balance the 2030 GDP burden of acute care costs of 8.5 percent between taxpayers and beneficiaries over time.[2] At present, the share is split 70/30 between taxpayers and beneficiaries, respectively. Should that balance change over time?

This chapter presents information that can be used in deciding who should pay and by what means. This question strikes at the heart of the current national debate on shared responsibilities vs. individual responsibilities. Issues of affordability and equity need to be considered in this context as well. Ultimately, the answer will be subjective.

Divided into four major parts, this chapter first examines ways to require beneficiaries to pay a greater share of the costs—by charging higher premiums, taxing benefits, or creating a defined-contribution approach. The second section considers ways to limit eligibility for the program, implicitly a way of making some individuals pay more for their health care. Third, taxpayers could be asked to bear a greater burden of Medicare through a variety of tax sources. Finally, the chapter examines issues to consider in deciding who should pay.

RAISING COSTS FOR BENEFICIARIES

One common option proffered for obtaining greater contributions from beneficiaries is to increase Medicare premiums. This increase can be done either across the board or by income level. (Greater cost sharing or limiting benefits, as discussed in chapter 6, are also possible, but going too far in that direction effectively negates the purpose of Medicare.) Another alternative is taxing Medicare benefits, which creates an income-related premium through the federal income tax system. Social Security benefits are already taxed in this way. Finally, a voucher approach could hold down the level of contributions per beneficiary, an option mainly aimed at controlling growth in spending over time. In this last approach, the initial savings are small but grow dramatically over time.

Substantially Increasing Medicare's Premium

Currently under Medicare, an enrollee is required to pay a premium equal to about 25 percent of the costs of Part B. Since Part B of Medicare constituted 47 percent of total Medicare reimbursements in 2004, enrollees effectively pay a premium of 9.4 percent of the combined value of Parts A and B of Medicare.[3] If that premium contribution were raised to cover 20 percent of these benefits—a figure comparable to that often proposed in health care reform options as individuals' contributions—the premium would need to be more than double its current level. That is, in 2005, the premium would have to be about $1,996 for the year—a $1,058 increase. If applied to all beneficiaries, this would raise almost $44 billion in additional premium revenues. In practice, the net saving to the federal government would be less, since those with very low incomes have these costs paid by Medicaid. Net federal savings would likely be about $41 billion after accounting for the increased federal Medicaid burdens.

Although this 20 percent premium would be consistent with employer-subsidized plans, Medicare benefits are also less comprehensive than those offered to younger families. So to achieve a more comprehensive insurance package, many Medicare beneficiaries pay all the costs for supplemental Medigap premiums or at least a share of premiums from employer-subsidized retiree insurance. Since premiums for Medigap plans tend to average about $1,800, Medicare beneficiaries in total are paying substantially higher premiums as a proportion of *total* insurance costs than those paid by many younger families. This is also likely to be true for most of those with subsidized employer coverage as well, since insurance burdens have been increasing over time. Further, when the drug benefit's costs are included, the Medicare combined B and D premiums will likely constitute about 12 percent of Medicare spending.

Although many Medicare beneficiaries could, without great difficulty, absorb modest increases in premium contributions, relying on higher premiums to "solve" a large portion of the financing problem for Medicare would create extraordinary cost burdens on moderate-income beneficiaries. If the Part B premiums were increased enough to capture 20 percent of Part A and B benefits, the total would be $1,996 in 2005. A single individual with an income at 150 percent of the federal poverty level (FPL; about $14,300 a year in 2005) would be paying 14 percent of his or her income for the Part B premium alone. Even at 200 percent of the FPL, the premium would still command over 10 percent of a beneficiary's income. When other costs of care from both Medicare cost sharing and noncovered services are added to this burden, most moderate-income Medicare enrollees would be routinely spending 30 percent or more of their incomes on health care. These burdens will consume an even larger share in the future since costs of care will rise over time relative to beneficiaries' incomes.

This level of burden often causes policymakers to consider creating an income-related premium in addition to an across-the-board increase. In fact, the 2003 Medicare Prescription Drug Improvement and Modernization Act (MMA) created a modest income-related premium. This new legislation, like most other income-related proposals that have been offered, adds a new premium on top of the existing Part B premium. It will be phased in for individuals with incomes above $80,000 ($160,000 for couples), eventually reaching a maximum of 80 percent of Part B costs for all persons above an even income cutoff of $200,000 for individuals and $400,000 for couples. Such a strategy allows the top premium to be much higher than the level feasible under a flat premium increase. This premium will begin in 2007 and be phased in over a five-year period. In 2011, when fully phased in, this premium is expected to shift about one-half of 1 percent of the federal government's cost of Medicare to higher-income beneficiaries (CBO 2004).

The challenge of an income-related premium increase is to find a politically acceptable change that recognizes both the need for reducing federal outlays on Medicare and the limited ability of many seniors to take on ever-greater health care burdens. If the limits where income-related burdens begin are set at a high level, they will raise few new revenues. It is estimated that the new Part B income-related premium in the MMA will affect only about 5 percent of beneficiaries, for example (CBO 2003). Substantial increases in revenues would require a lowered income cutoff affecting middle-income families, which would be less popular politically.

What is the appropriate point to begin increasing the premium? This question has no right answer. Mark Pauly (2004), for example, has proposed asking people earning 300 percent or 400 percent of FPL to begin paying more. This would affect individuals with incomes as low as $28,700 in 2005. Table 7.1 indicates the share of beneficiaries who would be affected by various income cutoff levels based on 2003 data. Because so few beneficiaries have high incomes, the cutoff level would have to be quite low to raise substantial revenues. For example, if the level at which people were asked to pay a higher premium began as low as $50,000 per year, only about 10 percent of beneficiaries would be tapped for a higher premium.

Further, the question of how high the income-related premium should be depends on where the threshold levels are set. If the thresholds are very high ($80,000 or $100,000 in income for a couple), then it is feasible to raise the share paid by beneficiaries to a higher level than if the thresholds affect those with more moderate incomes. Even

Table 7.1. Distribution of Per Capita Income of Persons Age 65 and Older

Annual income ($)	Percent earning (cumulative)
0–5,000	6 (6)
5,000–10,000	23 (29)
10,000–15,000	22 (51)
15,000–20,000	13 (64)
20,000–30,000	15 (79)
30,000–50,000	11 (90)
50,000–80,000	6 (96)
> 80,000	4 (100)

Source: American Institutes for Research calculations based on Current Population Survey (2004) http://www.bls.census.gov/cps/ads/sdata.htm.

when the initial starting point is set at a high income level, opponents of income-based premiums fear that the thresholds would be lowered over time.

The traditional way to think about an income-related premium is for one or a series of increases to be added at the top of the income distribution. An alternative would be to expand the Medicare Savings Programs which provide protections to those with low incomes, in concert with a general overall increase in the Part B premium. This alternative represents a different philosophical approach. The focus of the traditional income-related approach is on distinguishing between moderate- and high-income beneficiaries. An expanded Medicare Savings Program approach concentrates on protecting low-income beneficiaries from premium increases. Thus, its cutoff level could be set considerably lower, but the premium for those above the cutoff likely should also be modest. A combination of the two approaches is also possible.

Taxing the Value of Medicare Benefits

Another alternative for shifting the cost burden onto beneficiaries adjusted by level of income would be to treat Medicare benefits—all or in part—as income subject to the federal personal income tax. If, for example, half of the average value of benefits were added to the incomes of elderly and disabled persons, these benefits would be subject to tax rates that would vary according to other income received. This method would naturally result in a progressive tax on Medicare benefits. Taxing benefits is analogous to taxing Social Security, although it is more complicated because Medicare benefits are "in-kind" and beneficiaries do not traditionally view them as income. And although this approach could be added to the tax options below, since its impact is limited to beneficiaries, it is discussed here.

Not only would such a tax raise program revenue, it would make beneficiaries more acutely aware of the value of Medicare benefits and their growth rate over time. If only benefits for those whose incomes are above some threshold were taxed (as is the case with the taxation of Social Security), the extra burden would be restricted to high-income beneficiaries. This method could preserve universal eligibility for Medicare without a means test and still ensure that high-income elderly pay more.

How much would taxing Medicare benefits yield? The Congressional Budget Office (2005)—as part of its examination of revenue and spending options—has estimated the impact of such a proposal. For a beneficiary with an income above $34,000 ($44,000 for joint returns), 85 percent of the insurance value of Part A and 75 percent of the insurance value of Part B would be subject to income taxation. For single beneficiaries with incomes between $25,000 and $34,000 (and between $32,000 and $44,000 for couples), 50 percent of the insurance value of both Parts A and B would be taxed. Those with lower incomes would not be subject to taxation of Medicare. This option is structured in the same fashion as the current taxation of Social Security benefits.

CBO (2005) estimates new revenues to the federal government of $20 billion from this option in 2005. Over a five-year period (2006–2011), it would raise approximately $134 billion. The revenues from this option would rise rapidly over time since the income cutoffs are not assumed to be indexed to inflation. That would mean that a larger number of beneficiaries would be affected each year. In 2002, CBO estimated that a similar proposal would affect about 35 percent of beneficiaries (CBO 2002).

Taxing benefits would be a substantial change in policy, one that would make the program considerably more complex. Critics of this approach also argue that it is unfair to tax some in-kind benefits and not others. Consistent treatment of health benefits would lead to taxation of benefits from private employers, for example—another controversial policy discussed later in this chapter. Still, this option does offer a means for asking higher-income beneficiaries to contribute more without disenfranchising them entirely. And even if the amounts are only modest, such a policy (or an income-related premium) represents an important symbolic gesture of asking high-income seniors and persons with disabilities to pay more of the costs of their care.

A Defined-Contribution Approach

As with pensions, it has become fashionable to talk about changing Medicare from a defined-benefit to a defined-contribution program. That is, rather than guaranteeing, as Medicare currently does, a basic benefit package at whatever it costs to deliver such benefits, the government could instead establish an amount that it is willing to pay for each beneficiary. The contribution made for each individual would likely be adjusted by health status and by geographic location, but it would not be tied to the costs of a particular benefit package, especially over time.

The goal that unites most supporters of a defined-contribution approach is to reduce substantially the government's control over health care. Essentially, Medicare beneficiaries would be given a voucher to help pay the costs of the plan of their choice. The federal government would no longer act in the role of an insurer; traditional fee for service would be disbanded, and all beneficiaries would be required to choose among private plans. A key issue is whether beneficiaries would face a market much like the one that individuals under age 65 without employer-based coverage now face, or if new mechanisms would alter the market. The latter case would keep government more involved in health care to establish regulations on and oversight of insurance products, but it would ensure access to some type of standardized plans. Still, if the contribution were not high enough to purchase a good insurance policy, beneficiaries would have to pay more out of pocket.

Supporters of this defined-contribution approach believe that vouchers would make beneficiaries and insurers more conscious of costs. The advantages, from the perspective of voucher plan supporters, are the increased choice and competition that the market can foster, presumably resulting in higher-quality benefits at lower costs for beneficiaries. This approach assumes that economic principles would apply in their purest form. For example, individuals might be able to opt for larger deductibles or coinsurance in return for coverage of other services such as prescription drugs or long-term care. Since many Medicare enrollees now choose to supplement Medicare with private insurance, this approach would allow beneficiaries to combine the voucher with their own funds and buy one comprehensive plan. No longer would they have to worry about coordinating coverage between Medicare and their private supplemental plan. Persons with employer-provided supplemental coverage could remain in the health care plans they had as employees (assuming employers continue these plans). To the government, this option would have the appeal of enabling a predictable rate of growth in the program (Scandlen 2000).

But there are potential disadvantages for beneficiaries. Over time, the risks of higher costs of health care are borne by the beneficiary and not the government; the government's contribution presumably would be tied to a formula that may be unassociated with actual care costs. For example, the government contribution might be set to grow at the rate of growth of the economy, even if health care costs rise faster (as has historically been the case). In fact, the purpose of a voucher approach is to make the government's share a more predictable, stable amount, placing the beneficiary at risk for rising costs. But beneficiaries lack the clout of the federal government to obtain good prices. They would have to rely on competition in the private market to achieve any savings.

How successful is the private sector likely to be? As argued in chapter 6, the health care market is not as functional as many other markets for a number of reasons, including lack of good information, concentrations of market power, and geographic variability. The experience to date does not support the argument that private insurers would be able to sustain benefits over time without increasing premiums by more than GDP growth, for example. In addition, adjustments to protect the sickest and most vulnerable beneficiaries are not developed well enough to protect against adverse selection.

On balance, vouchers offer less in the way of guarantees for continued protection under Medicare. They are most appealing as a way to substantially cut the federal government's contributions to the plan indirectly, by eroding comprehensive coverage that the private sector offers, rather than as stated policy. The risks under such a plan would be borne by beneficiaries, which is of particular concern in an era when pensions and retiree health benefits from employers are less certain and Social Security benefits may be reduced. Retired persons' level of risk is increasing, and a key issue is whether it is advisable to shift even more risks onto individuals.

Savings from such an approach would not begin immediately since the voucher would likely initially be set close to the actual level of spending. Over time, however, a constrained rate of growth could yield substantial savings because of the cumulative effect of slower growth. For example, if a defined contribution were established that would allow per capita benefits to grow at 3 percent per year into the future beginning with the new drug benefit in 2006, per capita payments would average $13,454 in 2014, instead of the $15,663 level projected for that year (Boards of Trustees 2005). This reduced amount would represent a 14 percent decline in coverage—or an average increase in per capita liability of about $2,200 in that year. After 15 years, the gap would be 25 percent if the costs of the benefit rose on average 5 percent per year (as the actuaries have estimated through 2014), but payments only grow at 3 percent. Over time, substantial savings could be achieved but only by shifting the risks of higher out-of-pocket costs onto beneficiaries.

Pauly (2004) offers a modified voucher approach to allow Medicare contributions for higher-income beneficiaries to grow only with the general cost of living. He justifies his plan on the grounds that higher-income individuals should have to pay for the higher costs of technology over time. It is essentially a way to justify a limited growth rate for some of the beneficiary population. It has all the advantages and disadvantages of a voucher program, although it exempts those with lower incomes. Would such higher-income individuals be better able to overcome the obstacles to good care that a voucher imposes? The failure of the private market is still likely to be an important issue to overcome.

LIMITING ELIGIBILITY

Limiting eligibility for Medicare is implicitly another way to ask individuals to pay a greater share of their health care costs than if eligibility rules remained the same. Over time, increasing the age of eligibility, for example, would effectively raise the costs for all elderly beneficiaries, while options such as means-testing eligibility would differentially increase costs by level of income. Reducing the number of beneficiaries could generate substantial savings for the program, but each approach creates considerable problems.

Increasing the Age of Eligibility

The initial age of eligibility for Medicare could be increased over time. One of the justifications for such a change—aside from the primary one of saving the system money—is the increased life expectancy of the population. Since Medicare was introduced in 1966, life expectancy for persons ages 65 and older has increased by a little more than three years (CMS 2004a). As people live longer, they receive Medicare benefits for a greater share of their lifetimes. Increasing the age of eligibility could bring this proportion back closer to the level anticipated in 1965. In fact, Social Security has already adopted this approach for retirement benefits. The Social Security amendments of 1983 established a schedule by which the age of eligibility for full Social Security cash benefits will increase from age 65 to age 67 by the year 2027.

But the details are considerably more complicated for Medicare than for Social Security. Social Security allows partial eligibility at age 62. Medicare currently has no such provision. Many of those denied Medicare would face an imperfect private market for insurance that would require considerable reforms to meet the needs of those in their mid-60s. But such reforms have proven difficult to establish even after years of effort. Consequently, insurance costs in the individual market can be too high for even moderate-income persons to afford or can exclude those with various health conditions (Pollitz, Sorian, and Thomas 2001).

Without ensuring individuals the ability to obtain reasonable insurance, the number of uninsured persons would likely rise, exacerbating an important overall health care problem. Further, employers that offer insurance to fill in the gaps between retirement and eligibility for Medicare might drop that coverage, since this proposal would increase their costs substantially.

Perhaps most important, because this younger group is the healthiest among all beneficiaries, removing them from the risk pool produces only modest savings (Moon, Gage, and Evans 1997; Waidmann 1998). Almost 5 percent of Medicare beneficiaries are ages 65 and 66, and some of them would continue to be covered because they would qualify as disabled. Since spending on health care by nondisabled beneficiaries in their mid-60s is lower than that of older beneficiaries, this option would only reduce Medicare spending by about 2 percent once fully implemented. Moving too rapidly would create problems for people near retirement, those who have recently retired, and those who have made their financial plans based on outdated assumptions about Medicare coverage. Such a change would need to be phased in over time, so savings initially would be even smaller than 2 percent of Medicare's costs.

Finally, not all Americans are equally healthy at age 65. Life expectancy is increasing over time and the health of persons in each age range has improved, but not at the same rate. And while some Americans remain in the labor force or have generous retiree benefits at age 65, others struggle to make it to that age to qualify for Medicare. Many older persons who retire earlier or are moderately disabled at, for example, age 62 or 63, are in poor health and are poor candidates for purchasing insurance on their own.

To make this option less burdensome on those individuals, Medicare could change in other ways, allowing for at least partial eligibility for all those age 65 and above. This option could be analogous to early retirement benefits under Social Security, which are now available at age 62—an alternative that will be retained as the full retirement age rises, albeit with fewer benefits. Allowing people to buy into the Medicare program would address the issue of a poorly functioning private market, although it would likely mean that private insurers would enroll the healthy in this age group, leaving more expensive patients for Medicare. For example, eligibility might be retained at age 65 (or even lowered to age 62), but a higher premium (either fully recouping the actuarial costs or a portion of them) could be charged to enrollees until they reach age 67. In that way, Medicare would be available for those who must retire early. To offset risk selection effects of private plans and keep premiums at a reasonable level, Medicare might have to provide at least a partial subsidy and perhaps some low-income protections. Such adjustments would further reduce savings to the federal government, however.

Means Testing Medicare

The ultimate extension of income-related cost sharing is to make Medicare a means-tested program—available only to persons whose resources are below some specified limit. But, as was discussed in the proposal to raise the eligibility age, the private market would certainly not offer a reasonable alternative without further regulations. And in this case, those most disadvantaged would be the very old who have reasonable incomes but high health care costs. Again, higher-income elderly and disabled persons could be offered the option of either buying into the system at a nonsubsidized rate (such as is now done for persons over age 65 who are not eligible for Social Security benefits). Allowing a buy-in might be a more cost-effective approach for the government, since there might be savings generated from the economies of scale and low administrative costs of continuing to serve the full population, if no formal federal subsidy is involved.

The main justification for moving in the direction of means testing is to achieve budgetary savings. Advocates of a means-tested approach also argue that Medicare is not a sufficiently progressive program, since everyone eligible has access to the same benefits. However, it should be noted that although the financing for Medicare is roughly proportional, examining the combined effect of benefits and taxes does result in a program where higher-income beneficiaries pay a greater share of the costs (through payroll taxes assessed over their working lives). For example, an individual making $200,000 per year would contribute $5,800, and someone earning $20,000 per year would have a combined employee-employer contribution of $580 for the same insurance protection.

Another argument against means testing Medicare is political. Such a change would likely undermine the strong support for Medicare precisely because it is a universal program. It would constitute a major shift in philosophy from a universal to a "welfare"-based program. As discussed in chapter 2, the drafters of the legislation were very cognizant of what they were doing when they stipulated that the program include all of the elderly. They knew the political value of a program that would be viewed as a middle-class entitlement. So an income-related premium approach where some government subsidies remain is likely preferable to full means testing of Medicare.

RAISING REVENUES THROUGH THE TAX SYSTEM

Although policymakers and the public have largely avoided any discussion of increasing revenues to help fund the future of Medicare, it is essentially the elephant in the room that no one wants to recognize. The impetus for change has been almost exclusively in the other direction at the federal level in recent years—to lowering taxes. If Medicare is to remain without massive cuts in eligibility or benefits, additional revenues will be needed (Gluck and Moon 2000). Jonathan Oberlander (2003) documents a history of the willingness of taxpayers to provide additional funds for Medicare—both through general revenues and payroll taxes. Politicians, on the other hand, have been much less willing to raise taxes for this popular program, preferring to focus on various types of provider restrictions. Nonetheless, at least some revenues will be needed to balance out the contributions that will be expected from beneficiaries.

When looking for new revenues, the potential options differ substantially; the alternatives require a thorough airing. General revenue support, for example, will affect beneficiaries as well as younger taxpayers; the payroll tax is a well-accepted source of funding for these programs but largely exempts Medicare beneficiaries. The options below are not intended to be all-inclusive, but rather to suggest revenue sources that might be considered. For the most part, estimates are provided for 2007 and come from a recent Congressional Budget Office (2005) report on options for change. Because the 2006 estimates usually do not fully implement the changes, the numbers here are for 2007. To place them in perspective, the numbers are also expressed as a share of 2007 Medicare outlays for that year (estimated to be $371.4 billion net of premium contributions).

Increase Payroll Tax for Medicare Hospital Insurance

Payroll taxes, which now fund Part A of Medicare, could be increased either as part of a financing package or as the sole source of any needed revenue increase. While critics argue that an enormous increase in payroll taxes would be needed, it is important to remember that payroll taxes for Medicare start at a much lower level than for Social Security. A modest increase from 1.45 percent of earnings to 2 percent of earnings for both employers and employees would raise payroll taxes in 2007 to about $260 billion. The payroll tax share of GDP would go from 1.4 percent to 1.9 percent and remain there over time. This by itself would fully cover all Part A spending until nearly 2020 (Boards of Trustees 2005).

A larger increase in the tax to 2.5 percent of total payroll for both employers and employees would raise the Medicare payroll tax to about a 2.4 percent share of GDP—enough to reach past 2025. And in 2007 dollars, this would mean that payroll taxes would rise from $188 billion to $324 billion. This amount would exceed total Part A spending by about $116 billion in that year.[4] It is important to recognize, however, that payroll tax revenues are not expected to rise as rapidly as spending on Medicare—both because the share of the population receiving Medicare will grow faster than the taxpayer group and because per capita Medicare spending is expected to rise faster than per capita GDP.

Increase the Taxation of Social Security and Railroad Retirement Benefits

Currently, Social Security benefits are exempt from federal income taxes for single returns of less than $25,000 and joint returns below $32,000. Above those thresholds, benefits are taxed at 50 percent, rising to 85 percent above $34,000 for single returns and $44,000 for joint returns. The option of increasing the taxation of benefits would lower the thresholds at which up to 50 percent of benefits are subject to tax to $18,000 and $25,000 for single and joint returns, respectively, and lower the current-law thresholds at which up to 85 percent of benefits become subject to tax to $25,000 for single returns and $32,000 for joint returns. But although some of the taxes currently collected on Social Security go to the Part A trust fund, the concerns over Social Security's future would likely mean that there would be pressure for any new revenues to go toward improving Social Security's finances. Nonetheless, this option would increase revenues by $22.1 billion in 2007—or about 6 percent of Medicare's net outlays.

Tax as Income a Portion of the Value of Employer Contributions to Health Insurance

Currently, employees do not pay income or payroll taxes on income they receive in the form of employer-paid health insurance. As noted above, it is an option that would make sense in combination with taxing the actuarial value of Medicare benefits. CBO's (2005) option would treat as taxable income for employees any contributions that their employer makes for health insurance, plus health care costs, paid through cafeteria plans that together exceed $720 a month for family coverage and $310 a month for individual coverage. These amounts would be indexed over time to reflect increases in the general level of prices. In 2007, this would raise revenues by $30.3 billion from income taxes and payroll taxes. It would be a progressive tax both because it is part of the income tax system but also because these benefits are more heavily concentrated among higher-income workers. Like taxation of Medicare benefits, taxing contributions subjects income received in kind to taxation, something that is now rarely done. In addition, varying health care costs around the country make it difficult to design an equitable approach. The dollar amount needed to purchase comprehensive coverage differs and taxing in some places might therefore be considered too stringent. Finally, some or all of this tax could be reserved instead to help reduce the number of uninsured in the under-65 population.

Impose a 5 Percent Tax on Health Plan Premiums and Expenditures

Although many states have taxes on insurance premiums, there presently is no federal excise tax on insurance premiums or health plan contributions. This option would impose a federal excise tax of 5 percent on all health insurance premiums and expenditures for coverage under self-insured health plans. Payments to prepaid health coverage arrangements would be treated as premiums for this purpose. The tax would apply to related administrative services as well. The tax would not apply to expenditures under Medicare, Medicaid, or health plans for veterans or members of the armed forces. Such a tax is a mechanism for indirectly taxing the purchasers of health services. Moon, Segal, and Weiss (2000/2001) estimate that revenues for 2002 would have been 0.17 percent of GDP. That would translate into resources equivalent to about 7 percent of Medicare spending in that year. It could generally be expected to rise in tandem with Medicare costs, unlike many of the other tax proposals included here. This approach likely could be treated as an alternative to taxing the value of employer health contributions.

Increase the Excise Tax on Cigarettes and Other Tobacco Products

The advantage of a tax on tobacco products is that it can both raise revenues and discourage use of tobacco products. Its appeal is the relationship between smoking and health care costs. However, it is not an option likely to result in substantial revenue increases since these taxes currently do not raise substantial amounts of revenue for the federal government. States, on the other hand, raise considerable revenue from this source. The current federal tax is 39 cents per pack. An increase in the tobacco tax by 50 cents per pack would only raise 2007 revenues by $6.6 billion (CBO 2005). Further, such taxes tend to be regressive, falling heavily on low- and middle-income families, though studies show that such taxes do serve as a substantial deterrent to younger smokers.

Increase the Excise Tax on Distilled Spirits, Beer, and Wine

Like tobacco, alcohol creates costs to society, many of which are reflected in our health care system. Consequently, taxes on these products are often mentioned as a potential source of revenues to be dedicated to health care costs—in this case, Medicare.

The current federal excise tax on distilled spirits of $13.50 per proof gallon results in a tax of about 21 cents per ounce of alcohol. The current tax on beer of $18 per barrel results in a tax of about 10 cents per ounce of alcohol (assuming an alcoholic content for beer of 4.5 percent). The current tax on table wine of $1.07 per gallon results in a tax of about 8 cents per ounce of alcohol (assuming an average alcoholic content of 11 percent). This option would increase the excise tax to $16 per proof gallon for all alcoholic beverages, about 25 cents per ounce of alcohol. Tax rates would be indexed over time. One of the highest concerns for this tax (aside from its regressivity) is the fact that it would not raise substantial revenues. Revenues in 2007 are estimated to total just $5.5 billion (CBO 2005).

Together, the tobacco and alcohol taxes of $12.1 billion would pay for a little over 3 percent of 2007 Medicare spending. Over time, these revenues are likely to grow at a substantially slower pace than health care spending, thus falling as a share of Medicare costs.

Increase Taxes on Motor Fuels

Although current high gasoline prices may preclude a thorough discussion of raising the federal gasoline tax, this is an option that would encourage conservation and raise substantial sums. It could encourage companies to develop and promote other types of fuels for motor vehicles and discourage people from buying fuel-inefficient vehicles. Because of very high use of gasoline, small increases in the rate yield large revenues. Just a 12 percent per gallon increase in this tax (to 30.4 cents per gallon) would raise $16.8 billion in 2007 (4.5 percent of net outlays under Medicare) and over $181 billion across a 10-year period starting in 2006 (CBO 2005). Opposition to such a policy change would come from the regressive nature of this tax, as with other excise taxes. Also, it has differential geographic effects on drivers in the West and in rural areas. If this tax were to be used to help fund Medicare, it would mean a shift away from its dedication to the Highway Trust Fund. Again, revenues from this source would likely grow at a slower pace than Medicare.

Allow Some or All of the Income Tax Cuts to Expire as Scheduled or Earlier

Lowering income tax rates, changing the treatment of capital gains and dividends, and reducing the number of estates subject to the estate tax are examples of substantial tax cuts enacted since 2001. These cuts have already resulted in a substantial decline in federal revenues. The CBO (2005) has estimated that raising all income tax rates by 1 percentage point would increase revenue by $5.6 billion in 2007 and by $26.4 billion over the five-year period of 2006 to 2010. And if this change were limited to just the top two income tax rates on persons with the highest incomes, the 2007 amount would be $3.5 billion—almost 1 percent of Medicare spending. This last set of changes only partially reinstates earlier tax rate levels. For example, the top two rates of 36 and 39.6 percent from 2001 are now set at 33 and 35 percent, respectively. Returning these tax rates to their 2002 levels could raise $155.6 billion over the five years from 2006 to 2010.

A more substantial amount of revenues could be added to the federal Treasury by simply allowing the tax cuts of 2001 through 2003 to sunset as planned. Since a majority of these taxes fall on the well-to-do, many of whom will benefit from Medicare in the near future, it is appropriate to ask them to pay more before they retire. This approach also meets the concern of having higher contributions from those with greater resources. Reinstating just the income tax rates to their 2001 levels will retain $566.6 billion for the Treasury for the five years from 2011 to 2015 that could be used for Medicare (CBO 2005).

Further, most of the recent tax cuts will have benefited the same older persons who will benefit from rises in Medicare benefits. For example, higher-income elderly rely disproportionately on dividends and capital gains—taxes that have been substantially reduced. And the estate tax could be viewed as a way to tax decedents for some of the costs of their care at the end of their lives. Allowing these tax cuts to expire would more than cover the costs of the prescription drug benefit, at least for the near future.

Certainly to prevent these tax cuts from becoming permanent will be a difficult task. It may be possible to reinstate at least some of the taxes and dedicate them to Medicare, however. Such a plan would likely generate more support among the public than a simple reinstatement. In addition to estate and capital gains taxes, reinstating at least part of the reduction in general income tax rates at the upper end of the income distribution could be used in this way.

Institute a Value-Added or Retail Sales Tax

Under present law there is no national value-added tax (VAT) or retail sales tax, but most states and many local governments collect a retail sales tax. The option to impose a 5 percent VAT would add a new tax to the existing federal tax structure. The tax would not apply to housing, food, medical care, financial services, or education.[5]

In theory, a VAT and a retail sales tax fall on the same tax base: consumers. A comprehensive retail sales tax would impose a uniform tax on all business gross receipts from sales of goods and services to consumers. Sales to other businesses would not be taxed because the final product or service would be taxed at the retail level. In contrast, under a VAT, all businesses pay tax on their gross receipts. However, each business receives a deduction or credit for purchases from other businesses. Like the retail sales tax, the only sales actually bearing tax under the VAT are sales to consumers.

Each of the tax options raised above offers specific advantages and disadvantages. Either of the larger and more commonly cited options— the payroll tax and the VAT—could be used as the sole option for raising revenues. Other options, such as specific excise taxes on alcohol or tobacco, raise much smaller amounts of revenue. Two of the options, taxing the actuarial value of Medicare and reinstating the income tax, would be more progressive than the VAT and sales tax options.

Deciding How to Spread the Burdens of Medicare

From the examples presented here, it is safe to say that difficult choices lie ahead. And since it is unlikely that any one change will be sufficient to address the financing issues facing Medicare, a combination of options will likely be needed. A fair distribution of the burdens of financing Medicare also needs to be based on a number of considerations. First, as argued in chapter 2, Medicare is affordable from the perspective of the likely economic situation of the economy as a whole. Future workers, for example, will have higher standards of living, so increased contributions are possible. But the will to support tax increases needs to be there. Further, the decision should be an explicit one, weighing Medicare beneficiaries' and taxpayers' (some of whom are also Medicare beneficiaries) ability to pay. At this point in time, it is difficult to compare the abilities of future taxpayers to pay more to the abilities of future Medicare beneficiaries. In general, however, it would be safe to assume that living standards are less likely to rise as fast for those who are out of the labor force than for those who remain in the labor force. Estimates of the growth in Social Security benefits (even if they remain unchanged) indicate slower growth than in the incomes of the working population. In addition, it is likely that seniors and persons with disabilities will face rising costs of health care over time relative to their incomes. Certainly, they are unlikely to be able to absorb enough new per capita costs to avoid any more general tax increases and still sustain a viable Medicare program. While the current balance of 70/30 between younger taxpayers and beneficiaries of Medicare's costs might need to change, it is not clear whose relative burden should increase.

Simple comparisons of income levels between beneficiaries and younger taxpayers will not serve as an acceptable metric. A whole range of factors such as burdens on the young (of raising families and caring for children) and burdens on Medicare beneficiaries (of unusually high health care costs) need to be considered. And, the issue of perceptions of who can afford to pay will be key. Indeed, the definitions of high income or moderate income are usually not consistent when comparing cuts in benefits with higher taxes. For example, Medicare beneficiaries with incomes above $80,000 have been treated as well off while many politicians have justified tax rate reductions for those with incomes of $100,000 or more (Shapiro and Friedman 2004). Nonetheless, it is important to come to some consensus on a fair trade-off across options. It may make sense to pair tax increases with beneficiary contribution increases to spread the burdens of future financing.

In addition, other considerations are also relevant, including costs of administering new taxes, likely rates of growth of tax revenues over time, and whether earmarking taxes for specific purposes make them more acceptable. Some changes might be enacted soon but only introduced at a later time. Lessons from the 1983 Social Security Amendments may be useful to consider when deciding. Those changes were phased in over time and affected almost everyone in society. For example, increases in the normal retirement age passed in 1983 began to take effect in 2000 and will be phased in through 2027.

A summary of some of the alternatives described above and factors for consideration are shown in table 7.2. Because it is difficult to find consistent numbers and time frames for various estimates, the table contains likely revenues, premiums, or reductions in demands on Medicare as a share of spending in 2007. These estimates offer some orders of magnitude for further consideration. It is interesting to compare some of the examples. That is, raising the age of eligibility (and assuming for the moment it could be fully phased in by 2007) would constitute a major policy change but would reduce Medicare spending by only two-thirds as much as could be raised by taxing alcohol and tobacco (which as noted provides quite limited revenue increases). Taxing the actuarial value of Medicare is based on the same logic as taxing part of the value of employer contributions to health insurance. The Medicare option would raise about two-thirds as much as the employer contribution tax.

If the nation commits to Medicare and its future, we need to determine the level of funding and support needed to provide reasonable benefits to those eligible for the program, even if it means greater revenues. Broader views of financing and solvency than those com-

Table 7.2. Options for Financing Medicare

Specific financing or cost reduction option	Change as share of 2007 Medicare spending (%)	Additional comments
Increase the Part B premium to 20 percent of Parts A and B benefits with modest expansion of income-related premium	11	Most of the savings would come from the across-the-board increase unless the income limits now in place for income-related premium were lowered. Again, this is a cut in benefits.
Increase the payroll tax from 1.45 percent to 2 percent of payroll for both employees and employers	11	Payroll tax has not gone up for some time. This is the preferred tax by many tax-payers. A proportional tax that will not grow rapidly over time.
Tax the value of Medicare benefits for individuals with incomes beginning at $34,000 and $44,000 for couples	5	The income cutoff is not indexed, so the effects of this change over time affect more beneficiaries; thus it keeps up with Medicare growth over time. Has greater impact on higher-income beneficiaries.
Reinstate income tax rates to their 2001 levels in 2007 and remain at that level thereafter	5	Only a partial rollback of the tax cuts enacted in 2001 and 2002. This would be progressive. If limited to the top two rates, substantial savings could still be achieved.
Tax motor fuels by increasing federal tax by 12 cents per gallon	4	Likely to help with encouraging conservation but also would be very unpopular. Would create a new earmark.
Tax alcohol and tobacco as described in text	3	Tax is related to health issues; regressive and will not grow rapidly over time.
Raise the age of eligibility for Medicare to 67 (assuming full implementation by 2007)	2	Savings would likely be less in 2007 since more time would be allowed for phasing in such a change. This is effectively a cut in benefits.

Sources: Boards of Trustees (2005), CBO (2005), and author's estimates.

monly expressed today are needed in the debate on Medicare's future. According to the dictionary (Webster's 1966), a program is solvent if it is "meeting all financial responsibilities." If as a society we decide to support the Medicare program, we have the capability of doing so. If we view Medicare only as another expensive government program competing with all government services, the challenge is much greater. Hard choices will need to be made about what we want to support as a society. Revenues reclaimed by reducing fraud and abuse of the system and "efficiencies" from the private sector cannot provide the new revenues needed over time for Medicare. To serve one in every five Americans in 2025 will require substantial resources. Someone will have to pay more.

8

HOW SHOULD MEDICARE CHANGE?

Medicare is not a failed program, nor is it as unsustainable as some of its critics contend. For 40 years, it has provided nearly universal coverage to a vulnerable population group, changed with the times, and done a better job of constraining costs than has the private sector. This government health care program remains popular with its constituents. In fact, it fares better than private insurance in health insurance satisfaction polls (Davis et al. 2002). And although financing challenges exist, they are not insurmountable. Maintaining its success and the features that people value about the program should be paramount. These features include access to mainstream care, the pooling of risks, and additional aid to those in need. Without a strong government role, each of these would be difficult to maintain. From the perspective of Medicare beneficiaries, the goal of changes in Medicare should be to seek genuine efficiencies in the delivery of medical care, to ensure access to care for this population, particularly those with limited resources, and to find an equitable way to finance the program.

The inadequacy of the benefit package creates a number of problems, but this is not a failure of the program. Rather, it is a failure of policymakers to expand the program as needed. Some critics of Medicare suggest that past expansions of the program have scared taxpayers about the risks of any Medicare growth. There is no legitimate basis for this charge, however. The 2003 Medicare drug legislation, the Medicare Prescription Drug Improvement and Modernization Act (MMA), was the first major expansion in the basic benefits under the program and, as described in chapters 4 and 6, it neither fully covers drugs nor substantially relieves the overall out-of-pocket burdens facing beneficiaries. And there has been only one major increase in the population covered by Medicare, to persons with disabilities in 1972. Rather, costs have gone up with the costs of health care in general and with the growth in the population qualifying as aged or disabled.

How should changes in Medicare proceed? Just as was the case at its creation 40 years ago, the rationale holds to provide insurance against health care expenses and to fund such coverage for elderly and disabled persons largely through contributions by working-age individuals. The sharing of the risks of high health care costs has been a major accomplishment that the private market was—and still is—unable to provide. Uncertainty over future costs makes it difficult to determine how much to set aside if individuals were to try to pre-fund the program. Further, disability often occurs unexpectedly, making insurance protection for this group even more important. And finally, Americans as individuals have not proven to be farsighted financial planners; they are unlikely to save enough during their working years to fund these expenses at retirement.

New sources of revenue will need to be added—ideally before baby boomers retire so that they can contribute to a system that they will strain in the near future. Also, beneficiaries should bear some of the higher burdens themselves, depending on a reasonable assessment of their ability to pay. And within the beneficiary category, it will be important to distinguish between those with considerable resources and those who should face only modest increases in contributions. The income-related premium that is now a part of Medicare may be of more symbolic than financial value, but it likely makes sense to retain. The balance of who should pay will need to be recalibrated periodically as the financial status of beneficiaries versus taxpayers change over time.

It also makes sense to finance the program with contributions that bear a relationship to ability to pay. Although the payroll tax is not progressive, making all wages subject to the tax has resulted in what is effectively a proportional tax. The combination of taxes and benefits under Part A is progressive. Further, as Part B has increased in importance and when Part D is added, general revenues will be as important a share of funding as payroll taxes. While the payroll tax remains a stable and popular source of revenue, adding any new revenues might more appropriately rely on other sources.

Most Americans believe that basic health care is a right, and Medicare is now a well-established program offering basic access for nearly all elderly and disabled persons so long as they contributed during their working years and "played by the rules." At least for these population groups, universal coverage is well accepted. And universal coverage, in turn, offers a number of key advantages. This implies that the beneficiary base should largely remain the same, and not, for example, exclude those with higher incomes. Raising the age of eligibility might be an appropriate change, but *only* after substantial reforms in the private sector to ensure access to reasonable insurance policies in the private sector or if individuals are allowed to buy into the Medicare program.

Further, changes in Medicare that save federal dollars by shifting costs onto beneficiaries or reducing access to care do nothing about the overall burdens on society. Such shifting may hold down federal spending on health care for the elderly and disabled, but the need for care does not go away. One way or another, society will have to find ways to pay for health care or accept the costs of unmet needs and the resulting lower quality of life for the Medicare population. Discussions about the "unsustainability" of Medicare often conveniently omit this consequence. Saving dollars for the federal government is not the end of the story. Changes that simply shift costs, such as premium increases or raising the eligibility age, are more appropriately considered to be financing options and should be contrasted with tax increases in the debate over Medicare's future.

Most important, Medicare cannot function well if it is inappropriately restricted. Finding the right balance of comprehensive benefits, access to care, and sources of financing are important decisions for assuring a stable future for Medicare. These macro-level decisions are crucial to Medicare's future but unlikely to be resolved in the next few years. All of this requires recognition that an aging society will create challenges, but ones that can be managed. Addressing this sooner rather than later is important.

FACTORS CONSTRAINING MEDICARE REFORMS

Two challenging constraints place bounds on what can be achieved from Medicare in the foreseeable future. First, financing problems arising from both a history of high rates of health care spending growth (not unique to Medicare) and the long-run aging of the population put serious practical limits on future Medicare expansions. Over time, deeper funding streams will be essential, but the political climate precludes much if any reliance on new revenues at present. As a consequence, the range of possible options examined below for the near term is limited. The proposals made here should help position Medicare for the future; modest investments could pay dividends in the long run. But it is unwise to call for major expansions or reductions in the program until a more realistic debate on Medicare's future takes place.

Second, Medicare's place in the health care system needs to be recognized. Medicare cannot depend on cross-subsidies from other payers. Employers that help subsidize insurance for their workers became much more demanding in the 1990s, and payment levels to providers of care now are seldom generous from any source. Further, because Medicare represents such a large share of the market in many areas, it must offer reasonable levels of payment. That is, its size gives Medicare market clout and also increases its responsibility to the overall financial health of the system. Also at issue is how well Medicare can enforce certain changes if it is limited to just part of the health care system.

Practice guidelines or limits on ineffective treatments would be substantially more effective if done for the whole population. Since such activities need to change the attitudes of both providers and patients, efforts to influence practice should be viewed as system-wide changes for valid medical reasons and not just as a gimmick by one public program to hold down its own costs. Patients are more likely to accept constraints if equitably applied and based on evidence rather than singling out one group for second-class treatment. It may be easier to change attitudes of younger, healthier individuals in a broader reform than those of the typical Medicare beneficiary in any reform aiming to change incentives just among the Medicare population.

The absence of comprehensive health system reform does not mean that Medicare has to proceed independently of the rest of the health care system. A more coordinated effort is needed based on consensus among various payers about the right steps to take. The employer-based insurance market is now aggressively searching for ways to cut costs (Henry J. Kaiser Family Foundation and Health Research and Educational Trust [HRET] 2004). It has shifted away from putting pressure on health care providers to offer increasingly deep discounts as it did in the 1990s. And emphasis on strict managed-care approaches declined when patients pushed back on restrictions in the private sector. The latest approach by employers is to focus on raising employees' premiums, deductibles, and co-payments (Freudenheim 2004). Disease management programs and carve-outs for such services as mental health care are also part of the employers' strategy at present. It is possible that bold moves by employers, insurance companies, and managed care organizations may effectively begin to change the way that care is delivered. Medicare must be vigilant in adapting cost-saving innovations introduced into the private sector, including any changes in the overall delivery of care that may result from aggressive cost cutting across the board.

Even in the absence of comprehensive system reform, coordination between the public and private sectors can keep change consistent throughout the system—an essential consideration in avoiding cost shifts that do not necessarily save societal resources. Actively promoting better evidence on effectiveness and applying it to coverage decisions may be one way to achieve coordination. The information effectively is a public good that should be broadly shared. By investing only a fraction of its budget on such research and dissemination of findings, Medicare could lead this effort and be more efficient than many individual entities providing what may well be conflicting advice and restrictions on care. Medicare could be a leader in this area as it was in earlier years with payment reforms. Careful analysis and an investment in research by Medicare on delivery innovations could help convince other payers to respond as well. However, in too many instances of Centers for Medicare and Medicaid Services (CMS)–sponsored demonstrations, requirements for immediate cost savings often stand in the way of trying out new approaches or investing in research.

A major downside to aggressive cost cutting is an increased number of employers reducing their health insurance offerings. This could have important consequences for the Medicare program. Both early employer-subsidized retirement coverage before Medicare begins and supplemental coverage available after Medicare enrollment are shrinking (Henry J. Kaiser Family Foundation and Hewitt Associates 2004). Over time, this trend will increase Medicare costs if people lack insurance and delay procedures until they reach age 65. A recent survey by the Commonwealth Fund (Collins et al. 2005) found that one-third of people age 65 to 69 were uninsured before becoming eligible for Medicare.

Issues of fairness can and should be part of the debate. Medicare's visible position as a major publicly funded program can make it a target for cutbacks in spending. Yet tax breaks for employer-provided insurance also constitute a major—but more subtle—public subsidy. The public concern expressed over providing Medicare to millionaire seniors grabs many more headlines than tax breaks to corporate executives for very comprehensive insurance benefits. Medicare is more likely to be a target for change—perhaps unfairly—because it is such a visible government program.

These constraints combine to force hard choices for the future of Medicare. Overall, the lack of a clear consensus on any strategy for containing costs means that Medicare will require the attention and oversight of policymakers for a long time to come. This will, in turn, affect how much new financing will be needed and what changes to make in the immediate future. The crucial task is to identify which of those choices can improve the program, even in the face of cost constraints, and to avoid other choices that would negate the successes of Medicare.

FIRST STEPS

One set of productive changes, as outlined here, could be undertaken for Medicare without waiting for reforms elsewhere in the health care system. On balance, they would result in improved health care from society's perspective and likely generate some long-term system savings while only modestly increasing federal government spending initially. These potential changes include

- improving the fee-for-service portion of Medicare;
- improving the structure of the basic benefit package;
- expanding the Medicare savings programs;
- creating a new role for private managed care and establishing a level playing field between fee for service and managed care; and
- expanding the hospice program.

Improve Care in Fee-for-Service Medicare

A major challenge with facilitating better care for Medicare beneficiaries in the traditional part of the program is to retain the flexibility and choice that individuals now have but to offer mechanisms that can improve the coordination of care. Many of the demonstrations under way or planned by CMS to do so effectively put beneficiaries in a managed care–like environment (CMS 2004b). But managed care is what many of them wish to avoid by staying in traditional Medicare. Rather, it is essential to build on the notion of better information for both providers of care and for consumers.

Improving care in fee-for-service Medicare requires attention to ways to aid consumers in making good choices about care since they are in a less controlled environment, to provide mechanisms for physicians to serve as care coordinators, and to make coordination of care a less onerous task.

A key to better care is better knowledge about the effectiveness of medical care. It is difficult to expect patients to make good choices about health care without all the necessary tools to do so. Too often, "consumer-empowered care" is simply a euphemism for high levels of cost sharing. Information, however, is an essential piece of truly empowering consumers. Yet reliable information is hard to come by (or to distinguish from misinformation) and, in the absence of good information, many consumers are likely to use unnecessary services, increasing inefficiency in care delivery.

One place to begin would be with prescription drugs. Realistically, the new prescription drug benefit will require major efforts to hold down costs over time. Part of that effort needs to be based on evidence of the comparative effectiveness of various drugs, for example. Establishing rules for coverage of drugs should reflect good medical evidence with higher co-pays reserved for less effective drugs, for example, or brand-name drugs when equivalent generics are available. Too often, lower co-payments are established instead on the basis of which drug manufacturer offers the best discounts to the pharmacy benefits management company.

Undertaking these studies and evaluations represents a public good and should be funded on that basis. That is, such information needs to be comprehensive and reliable and shared with everyone. Only in that way can we change behavior. The debate on the prescription drug legislation called for such information. However, no funds were made available for such an effort in the legislation, and private plans and others are reluctant to do this on their own. Drug information should be just the first step in fostering better patient education.

Such support should not just be confined to consumers. Providers of care should also be brought into the effort. Many physicians, who have often resented the low pay in fee for service and the lack of control in managed care, would likely welcome the ability to spend more time with their patients. Surveys done for MedPAC (2003b), for example, found that one response to limited payments is for physicians to take on more patients and spend less time with each. But across-the-board payment increases do not represent an effective, targeted remedy. One possible way to change the dynamic would be to give beneficiaries a certificate that spells out the care consultation benefits to which they are entitled and allow them to designate a physician (or a team with nurse practitioners or physician assistants) who will provide those services. In that way, both the patient and the physician (who would receive an additional payment for the annual services and added staff) would know what care the physician is expected to provide. Where counseling on nutrition, drug coordination, and preventive services are needed, it makes sense to expand the scope of physicians by encouraging use of well-trained professionals like nurse practitioners who will spend time with patients. Such care would likely reduce confusion and unnecessary duplication of services that occur in a fee-for-service environment. Over time, this approach could help to control costs by reducing reliance on tests or referrals to specialists by busy physicians who do not have the time to spend with each patient to rule out simple problems or issues. Electronic medical records, with the appropriate controls on privacy, can also help patients who see a variety of physicians. Medicare could help to foster adoption of these records by setting standards and perhaps subsidizing their costs.

Revise Cost Sharing to Improve Benefit Package

A better balance and logic to Medicare's cost sharing could reduce the need for supplemental coverage. Rearranging the current benefit structure and asking certain beneficiaries to absorb higher costs might accomplish this goal within a reasonable budget. For example, costs could be kept low by modestly expanding the premium that individuals pay. Simultaneously, changes should be made in concert with expansions in low-income protections. In that way, low- and moderate-income beneficiaries could be shielded from higher premiums that would result from expanded benefits.

The most important adjustments in cost sharing should be combining the Part A and B deductibles and adding stop-loss protection as discussed in chapter 6.[1] Combining these two changes would lower costs for those with very high expenditures while increasing out-of-pocket costs modestly for people with lower spending. A reasonable combination could be chosen that would raise the share of expenditures covered by Medicare, offset in part by higher premiums. Consider, for example, a combined A/B deductible of $450 and a stop-loss of $3,000 (expressed in 2004 dollars). By paying about $15 per month in premiums, beneficiaries would have their cost sharing capped at $3,000. This would affect about 10 percent of beneficiaries. Another 14 percent would benefit from not having to pay the current hospital deductible, even though they do not reach the $3,000 stop-loss limit. About two-thirds of beneficiaries would face increased cost sharing of up to $350 each year.

Adding stop-loss protections and an improved A/B deductible would be unlikely to increase unnecessary use of services. Indeed, at present, cost-sharing mechanisms are essentially used to cut federal costs by shifting the burdens onto beneficiaries. And the beneficiaries who bear the greatest burdens at present are those with the most health problems. These costs particularly fall on those who do not purchase supplemental coverage and the very old for whom Medigap costs have become quite high. Those who decide to forego the high premium costs of Medigap (likely in the range of $1,600 per year) would have substantial savings to help defray any higher cost sharing they might face. The costs of coverage should fall even for those who keep their supplemental insurance.

There will also likely be calls for expanding the new prescription drug coverage since it leaves serious gaps in coverage. It is possible to design a benefit that better meets the needs of Medicare beneficiaries without expanding costs enormously. But the trade-off would likely be to move away from a voluntary benefit and make the coverage mandatory.[2] In that way, less attention would need to be paid to coverage for the first few thousand dollars of spending. As shown in chapter

6, the doughnut hole could be filled in and the coverage spread out to cover more effectively people at all levels of drug spending with very little increase in the cost of the benefit. And to the extent that there is attention to improvements in the 2003 Medicare drug law that would raise costs, the place to start should be with some of the aspects of the legislation that affect low-income beneficiaries.

Trends in private insurance coverage for younger families have increased cost-sharing requirements, making it easier to bring Medicare to a comparable level of protection. These changes in insurance comprehensiveness elsewhere help reduce people's expectations for Medicare, and even modest expansions could be effective over time in discouraging purchase of supplemental coverage. A reasonable stop-loss is an essential piece of improved coverage to effectively add catastrophic protection and ought to be high on the priority list for any Medicare changes.

Expand Low-Income Protections

Improved protection for those with low and moderate incomes should occur simultaneously with changes in cost sharing and premium increases so as not to put those with low incomes at a disadvantage. The hodgepodge of separate protections for the needy must be streamlined. The Qualified Medicare Beneficiary (QMB) program now pays the premiums, deductibles, and coinsurance of Medicare beneficiaries whose incomes are below the federal poverty level (FPL). Above that, the protection diminishes.

Cost-sharing burdens need to be lowered for more than just the poor. Those with modest incomes now have difficulty paying the premium and cost sharing, which can reduce their access to care. The new drug benefit offers slightly improved protection for people earning up to 150 percent of FPL. Expanding all the low-income programs to, for example, 175 percent of FPL and eliminating the asset test would represent a valuable investment in the most vulnerable beneficiaries. In 2003, more than 2.6 million people over the age of 65 had incomes between 150 and 175 percent of FPL, and CBO (2002) estimates that 1.8 million people with incomes below 150 percent of FPL will be ineligible for the MMA low-income protections because their assets are above the allowed limit. So at least another 4.4 million persons could become eligible for low-income support if these changes were made.[3]

The QMB program could be shifted out of Medicaid and the application forms streamlined. If done, this would reduce the welfare stigma and raise participation. A single supplemental program for low-income beneficiaries (aside from the Medicaid program) makes much more sense than the many confusing pieces that now exist. Many beneficiaries either are unaware of the program or are reluctant to apply for it through Medicaid. This shift would also help ease some of the pressures on Medicaid that will increase in the future with an aging population relying on that program for long-term care protection.

Level the Playing Field and Create a Unique Role for Managed Care

Although managed care under Medicare has lagged considerably below the growth in the private sector and participation declined from 2000 to 2003, it still serves 13 percent of all beneficiaries, more than 5 million people. In the interests of offering the same options to beneficiaries as are available to other age groups, it is important to retain a role for managed care within the Medicare program. Individuals who have had managed care coverage as workers and who wish to retain it should be able to do so. And plans that are innovative and contribute to improved health care should certainly be welcome.

But the new MMA goes overboard in its encouragement of private plans. There is no legitimate reason why plans should be paid 8 percent more than it would cost for beneficiaries who remain in traditional Medicare (Biles, Nicholas, and Cooper 2004). The more than $500 in additional per capita subsidies that this represents could, for example, fund generous stop-loss protection with no other changes in cost sharing for those in traditional Medicare if the playing field were level. Unless the subsidies available to traditional Medicare and to private plans are essentially equivalent, it will never be possible to truly compare managed care/private plans with traditional Medicare to determine which approach serves beneficiaries better and at a lower cost.

Further, more efforts to improve risk adjustment are essential not only to determine whether the playing field is level but also to create an atmosphere in which private plans could choose to take on the sickest beneficiaries and find ways to provide truly innovative care. The whole theory of managed care being able to better coordinate services should work best on those who need large numbers of services. Using private plans to develop innovations for multiple conditions with coordination of care would be a useful niche for managed care. Additional payments to encourage and reward such activities would not raise the same concerns as the extra subsidies do for the MMA. The new special needs plans of the MMA offer a promising start.

Expand the Hospice Program

Easing restrictions on the hospice program could make it a viable alternative to more aggressive types of treatment at the end of life at little additional cost to Medicare. Analyses generally indicate that hospice has saved the system money by giving individuals an alternative approach to end-of-life care and encouraging them to forego some of the expensive treatment they might otherwise receive. It has not been an expensive add-on benefit as many people had feared. In fact, a more important consideration is how to help this approach be viewed as mainstream care.

People view hospice as outside normal treatment, despite its considerable growth in recent years, and health care providers without the training and philosophy about end-of-life care too often avoid discussing its consequences and issues. Aggressive efforts should be made to educate patients and their families about alternatives and choices. Promotion of living wills and durable powers of attorney that allow Medicare enrollees to make their wishes known could be coordinated with these efforts. Too often, less aggressive care is treated as inferior care or even a withdrawal of support. Attitudes of patients, families, and providers about alternatives need to change. These educational efforts should focus on choice and not on requirements for limiting access to certain types of care.

Patients could be *encouraged* to participate in hospice care rather than required to have a doctor certify that the individual's life expectancy is just six months. Such certification is difficult for both patients and providers. Why not simply specify that the patient intends to focus on palliative care, recognizing that they have a terminal illness? Some resources could be spent to promote hospice care—for example, by funding demonstrations to stress that this is a reasonable choice and one that is easy for patients to make. Hospitals and other providers could be given financial incentives for providing space for hospice activities.

And for those who do not want to formally enroll in hospice, some services outside a hospice setting (such as counseling about end-of-life issues) ought to be available as well. It is in everyone's interest to encourage individuals to participate in planning such care.

Longer-Term Steps

The challenges in keeping the current Medicare program healthy into the future will occupy the attention of policymakers for years to come. Even if health care spending can be brought into line with the rate of growth of the gross domestic product (GDP), the aging of the population will likely necessitate both increases in the beneficiary contributions outlined above and additional contributions after 2010. Further restructuring of the program or adoption of private sector innovations may be appropriate over time as well. But for Medicare to remain a viable program, it will be essential to increase revenues from payroll or other broad-based taxes. Otherwise, it will not be possible to cover the growing share of the eligible population. Increasing service efficiency and effectiveness are important tasks that can help limit higher costs over time, but they are very unlikely to provide a solution. Implicitly, all of the other options facing Medicare represent financing issues; the question is who will pay and when. And if that decision is delayed for too long, it is possible that the quality of the Medicare program will deteriorate substantially over time with too much emphasis placed on unrealistic cost-saving goals. But neither is it necessary to make dramatic changes today given the uncertainty of future costs. A better strategy would be to establish a schedule of financing adjustments to be made periodically on the basis of 10-year projected costs and changes in relative economic well-being between the old and the young.

A Cautious Approach to Further Reform Medicare to Address Health Care Costs

It is just as harmful to make unnecessary cuts in Medicare as it is to ignore the need to make financing adjustments. A large number of uncertainties over health care service delivery and the private insurance market need to be resolved before it is clear what major steps need to be taken. If some of the reforms described above begin to slow Medicare growth to more reasonable levels, less restructuring or other changes might be needed over time. Despite claims by some that we have found the needed solutions to health care spending growth, experimentation and further modifications of new approaches are likely for some time to come. No magic bullets have been found yet; certainly putting one's faith solely in private market forces is a risky bet.

It is also important to distinguish which types of changes will actually slow the growth in health care spending and which will merely shift the cost burden to individuals and families. For example, vouchers can save money by limiting federal government liabilities under Medicare to a fixed per capita amount. But if vouchers do not lead to greater efficiency (by encouraging greater cost sensitivity by beneficiaries), then the problem of high costs will not be resolved; it will simply be passed on to individuals. Moving Medicare out of the public sector does not eliminate the problem; instead, it becomes only an indirect way to increase costs to beneficiaries. Further, the responses to vouchers will vary by ability to pay; higher-income people would pay a greater share of their incomes for care, but low- and modest-income people would likely have to make do with less care. Longer-term reform should keep in mind the importance of shared risk and equitable treatment that run counter to simply leaving the problem to beneficiaries to resolve.

Eliminate the Two-Year Waiting Period for Disability

One of the greatest gaps in coverage is the two-year waiting period that disability beneficiaries must endure before becoming eligible for Medicare benefits. Estimates indicate that there were about 1.2 million people in this waiting period in 2002 (Dale and Verdier 2003). While some of these individuals receive Medicaid protection or have employer-provided COBRA coverage (which makes employer coverage available at full cost to some former employees), an estimated 400,000 had no health insurance. Once someone has qualified as permanently and totally disabled, it makes no sense to delay access to good health care. Indeed, if future beneficiaries postpone care and their needs worsen over time, Medicare will still incur costs from that two-year waiting period. For quality-of-life purposes, this suggestion is a critical improvement in the program that should rank as a priority.

Increase Costs to Beneficiaries Where Appropriate

Passing further costs of the program on to beneficiaries needs to be carefully balanced against beneficiaries' ability to absorb these costs (and assessed in the context of such other benefit changes as those in Social Security). This balance can be analyzed in a relatively straightforward way for proposals such as increased premiums or cost sharing. Estimated per capita impacts can be compared with the income levels of the affected individuals. In addition, it will be important to contrast such changes with proposals that ask others to pay. Who is in a better position to absorb higher costs?

Raising the age for Medicare eligibility deserves a serious look in the context of the difficult choices the aging of the population will necessitate. But it comes with a number of disadvantages. First, without reform of the private insurance market, those out of the labor force may find it difficult to obtain insurance—and raising the eligibility age will increase the size of this vulnerable group. At a minimum, allowing older workers to buy into the Medicare program at reasonable actuarial levels would be important. A higher eligibility age would also burden employers that now offer retiree benefits, because they would have to fill in the insurance gaps for a longer period before Medicare eligibility would begin. Employers already face strong incentives to cut back on health benefits and have been doing so for many years. If, as a consequence of raising the eligibility age, the uninsured population rises, we will be just as burdened as a society as we were before. We will not have solved anything. The costs will simply not show up on the ledgers of the federal government.

Increase Public Financing for Medicare

Ultimately, covering Medicare's long-run costs will require additional public funds. Although the taxable base for Medicare has increased in recent years and some revenues from taxing Social Security benefits are bolstering the trust fund, Medicare will both implicitly (in the general revenue financing for Part B) and explicitly (from the payroll tax base of Part A) require further federal revenues, which is appropriate. The numbers of beneficiaries are expected to grow from about 14 percent of the population in 2000 to about 22 percent of the population in 2030 and even higher in later years. Both the share of GDP and of the federal budget devoted to Medicare *should* rise simply to keep pace with demographic change. At the same time, the share of the population with insurance from employers or former employers likely will fall, at least partially increasing costs to Medicare—a fact often ignored by those who talk about the unacceptably high level of spending on Medicare compared with the overall federal budget.

The payroll tax share of Medicare, at 2.9 percent of earnings (reflecting the combined employer and employee amounts), has not risen since 1986 (Board of Trustees 1996). It remains only a small part of the payroll tax total of 15.3 percent of payroll. If the percentage of payroll devoted to Medicare had been increased since 1986 by a factor just large enough to account for the growth in the share of the population who benefit from the program, the tax rate would need to be about 3.2 percent by 2000 and over 4 percent by 2020.

So even if Medicare were to achieve substantial savings in the provision of basic benefits, and even if beneficiaries were required to pay more, moderate increases in payroll or other taxes will need to occur. Such a revenue package for Medicare should include both new revenue sources from a broad taxpayer base and greater contributions from beneficiaries. The changes need to be undertaken simultaneously and adjusted periodically to reflect beneficiaries' and taxpayers' ability to pay to achieve a sense of fair treatment. A mix of progressive and dedicated taxes makes sense. For example, increasing income taxes on those with the highest income levels—and dedicating the revenues to Medicare—would ask high-income persons of all ages to contribute more to the program. Modest increases in premiums, the income-related premium, and other dedicated taxes such as payroll taxes and perhaps alcohol or tobacco taxes could further bolster the program. The types of changes suggested above do not imply allowing tax growth to "get out of hand." Rather, these changes should seem quite reasonable to the average taxpayer.

CONCLUSIONS

Beneficiaries' expectations for improving the Medicare program have declined since the first part of the 1990s. The failure to pass expanded health coverage for Americans in the 1990s and the current anti-tax, anti–big government sentiment militates against expansion. Indeed, much of our focus for the near future will continue to be on restraining growth in the program and perhaps even rolling back some of the drug benefits added in 2003. And many politicians will continue to claim that Medicare is unsustainable.

Changes can be made in the system, however. Improved cost-sharing requirements, some increase in premiums, better low-income protections, better information about and coordination of care, and an expanded hospice program are all worth undertaking. Indeed, it is crucial to seek these reforms rather than settle for cuts that only have budgetary goals.

The more difficult challenge is to make broader changes that could further improve the program. The problems of affordability of health services, the need to coordinate care better, and the importance of sharing the financing of care for retired and disabled persons will not go away simply because the population is aging. Over the next decade, Medicare will face extraordinary pressures for change, but the public should not assume that the only changes possible are declines in protection. Rather, this should be a time of considering how, as a society, we wish to adjust to the challenges and opportunities an aging society poses.

Appendix A

THE MECHANICS OF MEDICARE

The Medicare program was established by legislation in 1965 as Title XVIII of the Social Security Act and first went into effect on July 1, 1966.[1] In 2004, approximately 41.7 million persons were enrolled in the Medicare program. The program is traditionally divided into two parts: Part A is Hospital Insurance (also referred to as HI) and Part B is Supplementary Medical Insurance (also referred to as SMI). In 1997, Congress added a third part, Part C (previously referred to as the Medicare + Choice program, now Medicare Advantage), which is considered separately from the original fee-for-service Medicare program. In 2003, a prescription drug benefit was added with the passage the Medicare Prescription Drug, Improvement, and Modernization Act (MMA)—the largest benefit expansion in the program's history.

ELIGIBILITY

Medicare covers three groups of individuals: (1) persons age 65 and over who are also eligible for any type of Social Security benefit, (2) persons who have been receiving Social Security disability benefits for two years,[2] and (3) insured workers, their spouses, or children with end-stage renal disease (ESRD). Dependents and widows or widowers of retired workers are covered, so long as they are at least age 65. Disability coverage is limited to the covered worker or an adult disabled child of a covered worker. Eligible persons are enrolled in Medicare Part A at no charge.

About 86 percent of Medicare beneficiaries are in the first group noted above—age 65 or over. Medicare covers over 98 percent of all persons age 65 and over either as a worker or dependent. Anyone over age 65 who is not otherwise eligible may elect to enroll in Medicare by paying an actuarially fair premium. That premium was $375 per month in 2005. These are generally persons who have had little or no labor force attachment or who have immigrated to the United States from other countries and lived here for at least five years. Persons with substantial workforce experience—or persons married to, widowed from, or divorced from such an individual—but who do not have enough working quarters to fully qualify are entitled to a 45 percent reduction in Part A premiums. In 2005, this reduced premium was $206 per month.

People under age 65 make up about 14 percent of the Medicare population. The two-year waiting period for Medicare coverage for disabled persons, coupled with a five-month waiting period for eligibility for Social Security, means that individuals with disabilities do not receive Medicare coverage until 29 months after the onset of the disability. (People with amyotrophic lateral sclerosis [ALS] are waived from the two-year waiting period.) Disabled persons may continue to receive Medicare benefits for up to 36 months after Social Security cash benefits end, so long as they are still disabled. However, disability Medicare benefits may continue during a nine-month period of "trial work" and for up to 15 months thereafter. Persons disabled as children may also qualify for Medicare once they reach age 18 if their parents were eligible for Social Security. Dependents of disabled beneficiaries are not eligible for Medicare unless they are age 65 or older.

People with end-stage renal disease (ESRD) are covered once they file for benefits and if they are entitled to monthly Social Security benefits or are children or spouses of covered workers. In 2003, there were approximately 97,000 beneficiaries under age 65 with ESRD (and 94,000 age 65 and over) (Boards of Trustees 2004).

All persons enrolled in Part A of Medicare and all persons over age 65 may also elect to join Part B, which requires a monthly premium contribution ($88.50 in 2006) to pay some of the costs of the Part B benefits. (The premium is discussed in more detail under the section for Part B.) When persons enroll in Medicare or turn 65, the Part B premium is automatically deducted from their monthly Social Security check. Enrollees must inform the Social Security Administration if they do not want to enroll in Part B. If an eligible individual elects to delay joining Part B, a penalty (of 10 percent for each year of delay) is added to the premium to discourage individuals from joining only once they become sick.

The generosity of the federal subsidy means that most, but not all beneficiaries, join Part B. Most elderly beneficiaries elect this option, but a slightly smaller percentage of disabled persons do so. In 2004, among beneficiaries with Part A coverage, 96 percent of elderly and 88 percent of disabled beneficiaries elected Part B coverage.

Legislation in the 1980s made Medicare the secondary payer in cases where enrollees age 65 to 69 were still in the labor force and had employer-sponsored employee health insurance. The employee's insurance is liable for the bulk of acute-care expenses, and Medicare pays only for services not covered by this private insurance. This has since been expanded to include all elderly and disabled beneficiaries. Although this provision has been poorly enforced, in theory it limits eligibility for working enrollees. An individual may decline to take private coverage from an employer, for example, if a large premium contribution is required. In that case, the worker would receive full benefits from Medicare.

Yet another dimension of eligibility is the availability of the Medicare savings programs also known as the "Medicare/Medicaid buy-in programs," which assist low-income Medicare beneficiaries with out-of-pocket health care costs. Congress enacted the core part of these programs—the Qualified Medicare Beneficiary program (QMB)—as part of the Medicare Catastrophic Coverage Act (MCCA) of 1988, and although most of the MCCA was repealed in 1989, the QMB program remained. Under this program, all beneficiaries with incomes below 100 percent of the federal poverty level (FPL) and whose financial resources are under twice the amount specified for Supplemental Security Income are entitled to have the Medicaid program pick up the costs of Medicare's premium, deductibles, and coinsurance.[3]

These protections have been partially expanded into other eligibility categories within the Medicare savings program. The Omnibus Budget Reconciliation Act (OBRA) of 1990 introduced the Specified Low-Income Medicare Beneficiary (SLMB) program that has Medicaid cover Part B premiums for beneficiaries with incomes between 100 and 120 percent of FPL. A third program, the Qualifying Individuals-1 (QI-1) program, introduced in the Balanced Budget Act of 1997, was originally designed to cover Part B premiums for beneficiaries with incomes between 120 and 175 percent of FPL, but has since been leveled at 135 percent. In the QI-1 program, states may limit eligibility based on funding availability.

Although federal law defines these premium and cost-sharing assistance programs, states have discretion in how they implement these programs. Thus far, only a portion of those eligible for QMB or SLMB protections have signed up; many beneficiaries seem to be unaware of the programs.

BENEFITS

Medicare coverage is primarily limited to acute and post–acute care services. In general, Medicare does not cover long-term care services or all preventive medical care (such as routine physicals), but recently has begun covering a select number of screening and preventive services. With some exceptions, before 2006, Medicare's basic benefit package changed little since Medicare's inception.

Part A

Under Part A, hospital coverage is limited to 90 days within a "spell of illness," plus a one-time supply of 60 "lifetime reserve days" that can be used to extend the covered period within one or more spells of illness. The first 60 days of the spell of illness are fully covered (after payment of a deductible). After that, the beneficiary is liable for coinsurance for the next 30 days (a discussion of cost sharing follows). The lifetime reserve days, which would then begin, also require beneficiary cost sharing. A spell of illness begins when the patient receives hospital or extended care services and ends when 60 days have elapsed between such periods of treatment. Thus, a spell of illness is not really related to a particular illness, but rather refers to a period of time elapsing between discharge and readmission, when the next spell begins.[4]

Another Part A benefit is skilled nursing facility (SNF) care for up to 100 days in a qualified facility per spell of illness. This limited benefit must follow a three-day period of inpatient hospitalization and is restricted to enrollees who require the skills of technical or professional personnel for skilled nursing or rehabilitation. This is not a general nursing home benefit, but is intended to be an extension of acute-care treatment.

Hospice care was added to Part A as a benefit in 1983. It includes nursing care, physical and occupational therapy, medical social services, home health aide services, continuous home care if necessary, medical supplies, physicians' services, short-term inpatient care, and counseling. Persons electing hospice benefits face limitations on what other Medicare services are covered that relate to the terminal illness, however. For example, if a person elects to be in the hospice program, admission to a hospital is only permitted for alleviation of pain, respite care, or acute symptom management. Aggressive, curative treatment for the terminal illness is not covered. A physician must certify that the patient is terminally ill and is expected to die within six months, if the patient's illness follows the usual medical course. Beneficiaries are allowed two 90-day periods of hospice care and an unlimited number of

60-day periods. After the initial 90-day period, doctors must be recertify beneficiaries for hospice care at the start of subsequent periods.

Part B

Part B covers the services of physicians and other practitioners as well as a variety of medical and other health services not covered by Part A. In general, Part B of Medicare pays 80 percent of allowed charges after the enrollee meets a $124 deductible (in 2006). Covered physician services include surgery, consultations, home office and institutional visits, such as visits to patients in SNFs. Starting in 2005, Medicare covers a one-time initial wellness exam within six months of enrollment into Part B. It will also cover screening tests for early detection of risks for cardiovascular disease and diabetes. These are in addition to a number of preventive services such as mammograms and flu shots that have been added over the years. Coverage of services provided by certain non-physician providers of care such as dentists, chiropractors, and podiatrists are restricted. Mental health services are also limited to 62.5 percent of service costs. Other services Part B covers include x-ray and radiation therapy, ambulance services, physical and speech therapy, and rural health clinic services.

Home health, like SNF, is also a restricted benefit, but in this case is largely provided under Part B.[5] Coverage is limited to skilled nursing or rehabilitation benefits provided in the home. Unlike SNF, no prior hospitalization is required, and there is no limit on the number of days that can be covered. But home health services must be prescribed by a physician, with the expectation of rehabilitation for the patient. The care must be "intermittent," usually defined as less than daily, but recent guidelines permit a period of daily visits of up to eight hours per day. Finally, the patient must be considered "homebound"—generally confined to the home. The definition of "homebound" was relaxed in the 1990s to allow patients to leave the home for some short activities, including additional therapy, doctor appointments, and religious services.[6]

Part B also covers 80 percent of the reasonable charges for diagnostic tests, home dialysis supplies, durable medical equipment, artificial devices, and some outpatient drugs, usually administered in a physician's office (e.g., chemotherapy). Deductibles and coinsurance are waived for selected services, including mammography screening, influenza shots, and services provided in conjunction with a kidney donation.

Facility charges for hospital outpatient services and ambulatory surgery centers are also covered, again with coinsurance requirements. An individual treated by a physician in a hospital outpatient department, emergency room, or an ambulatory surgery center will receive at least two bills—one for the facility and one for the physician.

Medicare Advantage (Formerly Medicare + Choice)

The Balanced Budget Act of 1997 created the Medicare + Choice program, which allowed private sector organizations to provide medical coverage to Medicare beneficiaries in exchange for a monthly payment from the Medicare program. The Medicare + Choice program replaced Medicare's Risk Contract Program, which focused mostly on health maintenance organizations (HMOs), and allowed a variety of plans to contract with Medicare, including private fee-for-service plans. Under the 2003 MMA, Medicare + Choice was given the new name Medicare Advantage, again expanding the types of plans allowed to participate. For the first time, preferred provider organizations (PPOs) are allowed to offer coverage to Medicare beneficiaries.

Participating plans must provide all the services that Medicare covers. Beneficiaries who wish to participate must enroll in Part B and pay its premium. The plan may charge an additional premium in lieu of the deductibles and coinsurance amounts the beneficiary would pay if not in the plan. The plan premium may also be higher to cover services beyond what Medicare normally provides, such as dental care and prescription drug benefits. Both the frequency and the generosity of drug coverage declined between 1999 and 2003. For example, in 1999, 19 percent of Medicare + Choice enrollees were in plans with unlimited drug coverage—plans with no caps on drug spending—compared with 2 percent in 2003. Further, 44 percent of enrollees with drug coverage in their plan were limited to generics only in 2003 (CMS 2003). Those benefits are again expanding after the 2003 MMA changes.

Beneficiaries electing to enroll in Medicare Advantage must abide by the rules of the plan and will not be covered for any services performed outside the rules established by the plan, but they may disenroll once a year during the open season.

Plans participating in the Medicare Advantage program are at risk for the costs of providing health care to their Medicare enrollees. That is, Medicare pays plans a specified amount per beneficiary per month, but the plan is responsible for the cost of providing services to its enrolled beneficiaries. Thus, plans have a financial incentive to be efficient providers of health care. Plans are required to share at least part of any savings with beneficiaries in the form of improved benefits. Payments to plans were initially linked to average Medicare spending per beneficiary in the traditional fee-for-service portion of Medicare in the plan's county. Wide variation in spending among counties meant that managed care payments also varied widely. Because of this circumstance and because of market conditions, beneficiaries in some (mostly urban) areas have had access to plans offering greater benefits than those available to beneficiaries in other (mostly rural) areas. To address this inequity, Congress changed the payment mechanism when it created the Medicare+Choice program by establishing a floor rate for low-payment areas and limiting increases to plans in high-payment areas. In the Benefits Improvement and Protection Act of 2000 (BIPA), Congress raised the floor further. Despite these payment increases to plans, rural beneficiaries continued to have less access to managed care plans than their urban counterparts.[7] Changes made in the 2003 MMA may help redress some of these inequities. For example, plans are being encouraged to provide service to new Medicare regions that will encompass both urban and rural areas.

Enrollment in private risk plans rose rapidly throughout the 1990s, as shown in table A.1. Under the Medicare+Choice program, enrollment peaked at 6.4 million in 1999 (17 percent of all Medicare beneficiaries), and declined steadily to its 2003 level of 4.6 million beneficiaries (12 percent of all Medicare beneficiaries). The fall in enrollment was due to decreased participation from plans and beneficiaries since even when plans were available, lower benefits discouraged beneficiary enrollment.

To reverse this trend, the MMA changed the payment methods and further increased the level of payments to 107 percent of estimated costs for similar beneficiaries in fee-for-service Medicare. Plans are required by statute to use the additional funds to increase provider participation through higher payments, improve benefits, or maintain a stabilization fund to offset future increases in premiums or benefit cuts. Between 2004 and 2005, a substantial number of new plans have joined Medicare, including many which had earlier withdrawn from the program. Enrollment increased by more than 300,000 in HMOs and

Table A.1. Enrollment in Medicare+Choice (or Risk) Plans, 1994–2003

Year	Beneficiaries (in millions)
1994	2.3
1995	3.1
1996	4.1
1997	5.2
1998	6.1
1999	6.4
2000	6.3
2001	5.5
2002	4.9
2003	4.6

Source: MedPAC (2005).

by 80,000 in private fee-for-service plans between July 2004 and July 2005 (Gold and Harris 2005).

Prescription Drugs

Beginning in 2006, Medicare will cover the cost of beneficiaries' outpatient prescription drugs as an optional benefit under Part D. The MMA allows prescription drug benefits to be offered only through private insurers. Thus, for beneficiaries who choose to get all their benefits from private plans through Medicare Advantage, the drug benefit would be integrated into an overall package. But for those who opt to stay in traditional Medicare, a separate, standalone drug plan would provide drug benefits.

The new benefit will result in changes for those who currently have prescription drug coverage through other sources. Full benefit dual-eligibles will now receive prescription drug benefits through Medicare instead of Medicaid. Early information on this change indicates considerable disruption for those who are dually eligible. Medigap insurers will no longer be allowed to issue new plans that include drugs or supplement Part D coverage after 2006. Those who already have prescription drug coverage through Medigap will be able to keep those policies, but may face late enrollment penalties if they later shift to Part D.

Employers that provide drug coverage for their retirees have three options under the MMA. Employers can drop drug coverage for their retirees, in which case individuals could enroll in a Medicare drug plan or Medicare Advantage. Another option is for employers to provide wraparound coverage. That is, their retirees can enroll in a prescription drug plan or a Medicare Advantage plan to obtain the basic prescription drug benefit, and the employer can provide supplemental drug coverage to those retirees, although this would only push out the point at which the doughnut hole begins (when beneficiaries must pay out of pocket in order to reach the catastrophic protection level available in the Part D plan). Finally, employers could continue to provide drug coverage directly and receive a subsidy from Medicare. The overall benefit has to be at least as valuable as the basic Medicare benefit to qualify for a subsidy of 28 percent of each retiree's total drug spending in a given range (from $250 to $5,000 in 2006).

COST SHARING AND PREMIUMS

Enrollees in the Medicare program are required to share some of the costs of their own care—both through a premium for coverage under

Part B and payment of a portion of the costs of services received in the form of deductibles and coinsurance. Most of these contributions grow each year as health care costs increase under Medicare. All enrollees in the traditional fee-for-service program are liable for these payments, although Medicaid pays for certain low-income enrollees (described earlier in this appendix), and others may receive or purchase private insurance, such as Medigap, to cover these liabilities.

Part A

For Part A, cost sharing is organized around the concept of "spell of illness," as previously defined. Consequently, rather than an annual deductible, the deductible is assessed at the beginning of each spell of illness. If a patient is hospitalized several times during a spell of illness, only one deductible is assessed. On the other hand, if a patient has multiple spells of illness in any given year, several deductibles may be charged. The size of the deductible increases each year at the same rate as Medicare payments to hospitals. In 2006, the deductible was $952. The historical trends in this and other beneficiary cost sharing are shown in table A.2.

Similarly, coinsurance is assessed on the basis of the number of covered days during a spell of illness. (The calculation of number of days may cumulate across multiple admissions to the hospital.) The first 60 days of hospital care require no coinsurance. Between days 61 and 90 of the spell, the individual is assessed coinsurance of one-fourth the hospital deductible for each day (or $238 in 2006). After 90 days of hospitalization during a spell of illness, the Medicare beneficiary must draw upon a lifetime reserve of 60 additional days of coverage while paying coinsurance equal to one-half the deductible ($476 in 2006) for each day. After exhausting that reserve, the Medicare beneficiary is liable for the full costs of any additional days in the hospital. About 0.5 percent of all Medicare enrollees exhaust their lifetime reserve days in any one year, usually because they have experienced multiple hospitalizations.

Coinsurance is also assessed on days 21 through 100 of a skilled nursing facility stay. The amount is set at one-eighth of the hospital deductible. At $119 in 2006, this amount averages about half of what Medicare pays SNFs per day.[8] Consequently, many beneficiaries simply do not receive SNF care for more than 20 days per spell of illness.

In addition to the hospital deductible, there is another deductible equal to the cost of the first three pints of whole blood a beneficiary receives as part of covered inpatient services. This deductible is also calculated on a spell-of-illness basis. The patient can avoid this deductible by arranging for replacement of the blood by donors.

Table A.2. Medicare Deductibles, Coinsurance, and Premiums, 1966–2005

For benefit periods beginning in calendar year	Inpatient Hospital			Skilled nursing facility, 21st through 100th-day coinsurance ($)	Supplementary Medical Insurance deductible ($)	Supplementary Medical Insurance premium ($)
	First 60 days' deductible ($)	61st through 90th day, coinsurance per day ($)	60 lifetime reserve days ($)			
1966	40	10	—	—	50	3.00
1967	40	10	—	5.00	50	3.00
1968	40	10	20	5.00	50	4.00
1969	44	11	22	5.50	50	4.00
1970	52	13	26	6.50	50	5.30
1971	60	15	30	7.50	50	5.60
1972	68	17	34	8.50	50	5.80
1973	72	18	36	9.00	60	6.30
1974	84	21	42	10.50	60	6.70
1975	92	23	46	11.50	60	6.70
1976	104	26	52	13.00	60	7.20
1977	124	31	62	15.50	60	7.70
1978	144	36	72	18.00	60	8.20
1979	160	40	80	20.00	60	8.70
1980	180	45	90	22.50	60	9.60
1981	204	51	102	25.50	60	11.00
1982	260	65	130	32.50	75	12.20
1983	304	76	152	38.00	75	12.20
1984	356	89	178	44.50	75	14.60
1985	400	100	200	50.00	75	15.50
1986	492	123	246	61.50	75	15.50
1987	520	130	260	65.00	75	17.90
1988	540	135	270	67.50	75	24.80
1989[a]	560	n.a.	n.a.	25.50	75	31.90
1990	592	148	296	74.00	75	28.60
1991	628	157	314	78.50	100	29.90
1992	652	163	326	81.50	100	31.80
1993	676	169	338	84.50	100	36.60
1994	696	174	348	87.00	100	41.10
1995	716	179	358	89.50	100	46.10
1996	736	184	368	92.00	100	42.50
1997	760	190	380	95.00	100	13.80
1998	764	191	382	95.50	100	43.80
1999	768	192	384	96.00	100	45.50
2000	776	194	388	97.00	100	45.50
2001	792	198	396	99.00	100	50.00
2002	812	203	406	101.50	100	54.00
2003	840	210	420	105.00	100	58.70
2004	876	219	438	109.50	100	66.60
2005	912	228	456	114.00	110	78.10

Source: Boards of Trustees (2005).
[a] Includes MCCA legislation.
n.a. = not applicable

Finally, the hospice program requires two coinsurance payments. Beneficiaries must pay 5 percent coinsurance (not to exceed $5) for each palliative drug and biological prescription furnished by the hospice when the beneficiary is not an inpatient. A 5 percent coinsurance payment is also required for each day of respite care (maximum five days), capped at the level of the hospital deductible.

Part B

Under Part B, the deductible was $124 in 2006. Until recently, the premium did not rise automatically over time and was increased only three times by legislation from an initial level of $50 per year. The MMA increased the deductible for a fourth time to $110 per year beginning in 2005, and now rises by the annual percentage increase in Part B spending each year. For physician and certain other services, the coinsurance is set at 20 percent of the amount that Medicare establishes as its "allowed" charge. Two major exceptions to the coinsurance requirement are clinical laboratory services, for which Medicare usually reimburses 100 percent of the fee schedule, and home health services. A 20 percent coinsurance payment was required for home health until 1973. Coinsurance does apply to some items supplied through home health care, such as durable medical equipment (DME). Most other services under Part B are subject to the coinsurance requirement. Since Part B payments generally rise each year, the amount that Medicare beneficiaries pay in cost sharing consequently goes up even when the same level of services is used from year to year.

The Part B premium is also tied to the costs of Part B services. Enrollees must pay approximately 25 percent of the costs of care for an elderly enrollee. That amount was first introduced as a temporary change in 1982 and was periodically extended on an ad hoc basis. For a period in the early 1990s, the premiums were established by legislation, in anticipation of higher physician costs after adoption of the new physician fee schedule. Consequently, in 1995, premiums covered about 31.5 percent of Part B costs. In 1996, this share returned to 25 percent of costs and has since remained at that level. In 1997, the Balanced Budget Act permanently set the Part B premium at 25 percent. The monthly premium in 2006 is $88.50.

The original share that enrollees paid was higher, set at 50 percent in the enacting legislation. But over time, the premium grew much faster than Social Security payments, resulting in a Part B premium deduction from Social Security that was consuming an ever-increasing portion of monthly Social Security checks. The 1972 amendments to Medicare changed the premium so that thereafter it would grow no faster than the rate of the Social Security cost-of-living adjustment

(COLA). Then the reverse problem arose. With high rates of health care spending in the 1970s, the share beneficiaries paid gradually eroded to about 25 percent of Part B costs by 1981. The 1981 legislation essentially froze the premium share at 25 percent of the costs of an elderly enrollee as a federal budget reduction measure.

Normally, the premium is automatically deducted from the beneficiary's Social Security check. Each January, both the Social Security COLA and the premium increase go into effect. An additional protection for beneficiaries with small monthly payment amounts is that for each enrollee, the Part B premium is not allowed to rise (in dollars) by an amount greater than the Social Security COLA. Consequently, where the increase in Part B premiums effectively eliminates a few enrollees' COLA each year, no one actually receives less in nominal dollars from one year to the next because of Medicare premium increases. And in practice, unless the Social Security COLA is very small and the Part B premium increase very large, only a few beneficiaries have their full COLA eliminated.

Traditionally, beneficiaries paid the same Part B premiums regardless of income or assets. Beginning in 2007, a change will be phased in that will require single individuals with incomes over $80,000 ($160,000 for couples) to pay higher Part B premiums. This change is estimated initially to affect 1.2 million beneficiaries, but will rise over time since the income cutoffs are not indexed.

Medicare Advantage

As mentioned previously, plans may charge premiums in lieu of Part B cost sharing, or for extra non-Medicare-covered benefits. The share of Medicare + Choice plans charging premiums increased steadily from 15 percent in 1999 to 62 percent in 2003 (CMS 2004a). Further, average monthly Medicare + Choice premiums increased from $5.35 in 1999 to $37 in 2003. Overall, cost sharing also increased for beneficiaries enrolled in the program, with particular increases in co-payments for physician visits and inpatient hospitalizations. In 2001, only 4 percent of enrollees had over $50 in monthly cost-sharing payments, increasing to 14 percent in 2003 (CMS 2004a).

The higher payments for Medicare Advantage plans that began in 2004 are expected to reverse the trend for ever-higher beneficiary burdens, at least for the next several years. Early information suggests that the higher payments have been divided between improved benefits (and hence lower cost sharing) and higher payments to service providers.

Prescription Drugs

Those who stay in traditional Medicare and enroll in Part D will pay a monthly premium averaging $32 per month in 2006. Projections indicate that the premium will likely rise to $58 per month by 2013. Beneficiaries who delay enrollment past the initial period will be assessed financial penalties, with premiums rising at least 1 percent for each month of delay.

Under the standard benefit, individuals have to meet a deductible of $250 before the government pays any benefits. For drug spending between $251 and $2,250, the plan pays for 75 percent of the costs. Individuals are then responsible for all drug costs from $2,251 until they have spent $3,600 out of pocket. This will occur when total spending reaches $5,100. At that point, the beneficiary reaches the catastrophic limit and pays just 5 percent of prescription drug costs. These thresholds are indexed to grow annually by the growth in per capita Part D spending of Medicare beneficiaries. Unlike the Part B premium, there are no guarantees that Part D premiums will be limited to the dollar increase in the yearly Social Security COLA.

Premium and cost-sharing assistance is available to those with low incomes and limited assets. Medicaid full benefit dual eligibles with incomes below 100 percent of FPL will receive a full premium subsidy, not be required to pay a deductible, and have cost sharing of just $1 for generic and $3 for brand-name drugs. Medicaid beneficiaries above the poverty level and non-Medicaid beneficiaries with incomes below 135 percent of FPL (and who meet the asset requirement) will have slightly higher co-pays. Other enrollees with incomes between 135 and 150 percent of FPL and who meet certain asset tests are eligible for sliding scale premium subsidies, a $50 deductible, and reduced levels of cost sharing on prescription drugs. In the first few weeks of this program, these low-income protections have not always been honored for low-income beneficiaries (Connolly 2006).

Growth in Fee-for-Service Enrollee Liability

Since most of the cost sharing under Medicare is linked to expenditures, enrollees' liabilities have risen sharply over time. Most of the liability in the traditional fee-for-service program comes from Part B, through coinsurance and the premium. Together, they constitute three-fourths of Medicare's cost sharing (on services covered before prescription drugs were added). Thus, although Part B is less expensive from the standpoint of federal dollars, it is the more costly program as far as beneficiaries are concerned. In 2004, Part B constituted about 39 percent of federal spending on Parts A and B combined. In general, cost sharing by any insurer, including Medicare, is seen as a mechanism for preventing beneficiaries from overusing health care services. Acute hospital admissions—arguably less discretionary than Part B services—have lower beneficiary cost sharing but constitute the bulk of Medicare spending.

Beneficiaries may be asked by their physicians to pay in full at the time of service, although physicians are required to file for reimbursement on beneficiaries' behalf.[9] Physicians who directly bill Medicare are said to "accept assignment." If they accept assignment for all their Medicare patients, they are termed "participating providers" and are eligible for somewhat higher payments (allowed charges) for services. This financial incentive was made to encourage physicians to take assignment. If physicians decline to take assignment, they deal directly with the patient, who then must be reimbursed by Medicare. When such physicians bill their patients for more than the allowed charges, they are said to "balance bill" the patients, effectively asking patients to pay more than the formal coinsurance of 20 percent of allowed charges. Beginning in 1993, physicians are allowed to charge no more than 115 percent of their approved charges, limiting any balance billing. The number of physicians seeking to balance bill their patients has declined dramatically over time. Average annual beneficiary liability for balance billing grew from $56 in 1980 to a high of $88 in 1986, and has since fallen to $3 in 1999. The extent of balance billing varies by location of practice and specialty, however.

Physicians may refuse to abide by these limits. If they do, the Medicare program does not cover their charges and beneficiaries are liable for the full amount of the physician's charge. Most physicians have continued to abide by these rules and accept Medicare patients.

PAYING PROVIDERS

In all, Medicare pays for health care services using 15 payment systems generally organized by the setting in which care is received. The 15 payment systems are for acute care hospitals, ambulance services, ambulatory surgical centers, durable medical equipment, home health care, hospice care, hospital outpatient departments, inpatient rehabilitation facilities, long-term care hospitals, outpatient dialysis, outpatient laboratories, physician care, psychiatric facilities, skilled nursing facilities, and Medicare Advantage plans.

The payment policies and methods are extremely complex and have evolved over time. In the traditional fee-for-service (FFS) program, Medicare sets the payment amounts that providers will receive for most covered products and services. When beneficiaries use services, providers submit bills to Medicare and collect beneficiary coinsurance as applicable. In the Medicare Advantage program, as described earlier, monthly predetermined payments are made automatically to health plans, regardless of the services enrolled beneficiaries use. Although hospitals and other major providers in the fee-for-service program are paid according to the services they provide, they do not file each claim separately. Rather, they are paid periodically, with adjustments to reconcile the actual amounts they are owed.[10]

Initially, payment policy for hospitals and other large providers was based simply on reported costs. In the case of physicians, for example, payments reflected "reasonable charges," defined as the lower of either a physician's own usual or customary charge, or the prevailing charge for physicians in a particular area. Then, as Medicare spending began steeply increasing, measures to control costs were incorporated into Medicare's payment systems, fundamentally changing the way Medicare pays for many products and services. For example, prospective payment systems, which establish fixed payments meant to cover a bundle of services, have been implemented in most of Medicare's major payment systems, with many being instituted in legislation between 1983 and 1997. The most well known is the prospective payment system for hospitals, which pays on the basis of a particular diagnosis regardless of the specific care a patient receives (unless the length of stay is so high as to trigger an "outlier" payment).

Since 1992, Medicare has paid physicians based on the Medicare fee schedule, which lists the relative amount that Medicare will pay for more than 7,000 physician services. Each year a base dollar amount is set and then multiplied against each of the relative fee levels to determine the actual payment. For many services, Medicare payments can be higher when physicians provide them in an office setting than when the same service is provided in a facility, such as a hospital, to account for the overhead costs (practice expenses) physicians incur for supplying and maintaining their office environment. When the service is provided in a facility, Medicare pays both the facility and the physician. As discussed earlier, physicians who are participating providers are eligible for higher payments than physicians who bill their patient directly and seek balance billing.

FINANCING THE MEDICARE PROGRAM

Medicare Part A is financed almost entirely by a 1.45 percent tax on earnings, assessed on both employees and employers (and thus is a 2.9 percent tax on overall payroll). It is part of the Federal Insurance Contributions Act (FICA) tax that most individuals see as a deduction in their paychecks each pay period. It is assessed regardless of wage level on persons of all ages, but is paid mostly by persons under age 65 (since few persons over that age remain in the labor force). Medicare now differs from Social Security because there is no limit on earnings subject to Medicare's tax; while in 2005, Social Security's payroll tax applied to only the first $95,000 of a worker's earnings. The Medicare payroll tax *rate* was last increased in 1986 as part of the 1983 Social Security amendments and is not currently scheduled to rise further.

In 1966, the initial tax rate was 0.7 percent (combined) against a base of $6,600 in earnings—or a maximum contribution of $46.20 per person that year. Today, there is effectively no limit since all earnings are subject to the tax. A worker with earnings of $200,000 in a given year, for example, would have a total contribution (from both employee and employer contributions) of $5,800. A worker earning $30,000 in a given year would have a total contribution of $870.

These revenues are combined with premiums (paid by those elderly not otherwise eligible for Part A), part of the taxation of Social Security benefits, small general revenue transfers to cover beneficiaries such as railroad retirees, and interest from previous balances in the Trust Fund to form the Federal Hospital Insurance Trust Fund. Under the law, payments are made only so long as there is a positive balance in the trust fund. The HI Trustees report for 2005 indicates a declining balance in the near term to 89 percent of Part A spending in 2013, as listed in table A.3, and total exhaustion of the trust fund by 2019.

Table A.3. Estimated Operations of Federal Hospital Insurance Trust Fund, 1998–2009 ($ billions)

Calendar year	Total income (billing $)	Total disbursements ($)	Net increase in fund ($)	Fund at end of year ($)
2003	175.8	154.6	21.2	256.0
2004	183.9	170.6	13.3	269.3
2005	195.0	182.5	12.5	281.8
2006	191.6	194.5	12.0	293.8
2007	218.4	208.0	10.5	304.3
2008	230.6	219.4	11.3	315.6
2009	242.7	233.3	9.4	325.0
2010	254.3	248.5	5.9	330.8
2011	268.0	264.8	3.2	334.0
2012	281.9	283.2	−1.3	332.8
2013	295.3	299.8	−7.9	324.8
2014	308.4	323.9	−15.5	309.3

Source: Boards of Trustees (2005).

Note: Data are based on alternative II assumptions, which are usually considered intermediate asssumptions regarding factors such as life expectancy and health care inflation.

Part B's funding comes from the premium contributions of beneficiaries and general revenue contributions by the federal government. Although there is a trust fund for Part B, as well as Part A, it is much less important since, by law, the U.S. Treasury must make up the difference between premium contributions and Part B spending. Thus, while general revenue contributions may be large, there is no crisis in funding requiring legislation as there is with Part A. But Part B's growth has actually been higher than that for Part A in recent years, raising financing concerns for this part of Medicare as well. As a consequence, the MMA established a new measure of fiscal solvency based on the share of Medicare spending coming from general revenues. Once general revenues (essentially defined as the residual left after subtracting dedicated revenues from total Medicare spending in each year) are projected to reach 45 percent of total spending within the next seven years, a warning would be generated, presumably encouraging federal legislation to curb spending on Medicare. Such a warning may occur as early as 2006.

The new Part D benefit will be funded in a manner similar to the way Part B is funded. Beneficiaries choosing to enroll in Part D will pay a premium set to cover 25 percent of the costs of the benefits, with the balance coming from general revenues. In practice, general revenues will be greater than 75 percent of the costs of the benefit since subsidies for those with low incomes must also be covered. Initially, states will be required to pay a large share of those subsidies. Over time, the state contributions will decline and general revenues will be tapped to pay increasingly for these low-income subsidies. This will also affect the general revenue funding measure that has been added to the trust fund reports.

ADMINISTERING THE MEDICARE PROGRAM

The Centers for Medicare and Medicaid Services (CMS), formerly the Health Care Financing Administration (HCFA), is in charge of overseeing the Medicare program and promulgates rules and regulations governing its operations. The administrative costs of the program are quite low overall—less than 2 percent of program outlays. Day-to-day processing of claims and oversight of providers is done at a much more disaggregated level, however. CMS contracts with "fiscal intermediaries" to process Part A claims and contracts with "carriers" to process Part B claims. These groups, usually insurance companies, deal directly with hospitals and physicians, respectively, to determine the appropriate levels of payment and then pay those providers. These entities also check claims for accuracy and fraud, and provide summary records of health care use to CMS.

Carriers and intermediaries have always had considerable latitude in interpreting CMS instructions, often resulting in inconsistent enforcement of regulations. In recent years, however, CMS has improved its data management and has gradually increased its ability to oversee the work of the carriers and intermediaries. Medicare also pays providers in a timely fashion—often at a faster rate than that of private insurers. For example, CMS has initiated policies requiring carriers to meet more uniform reporting requirements. CMS has also improved its data collection and reporting systems, increasing the timeliness and usefulness of the data. Two-year lag times in data collection and release are common, and mark an improvement from earlier processing times.

CMS contracts with Quality Improvement Organizations (QIOs) to improve the overall level of quality beneficiaries receive, particularly in hospitals. The QIO program has resulted in the development of numerous quality measures and an infrastructure to assist providers, such as hospitals and SNFs, with technical help in designing quality improvement programs. QIOs are also required to work on complaints and appeals. This part of their activities will likely expand further over time as they deal with the new Part D drug benefit.

The MMA legislation has also added a new Office of the Medicare Ombudsman to the administrative functions of CMS. This office will largely collect information and data from other sources, including QIOs, state health counseling programs, carriers, and intermediaries. The goal is to centralize customer service and identification of problems that beneficiaries face.

CMS also addresses quality concerns through its recent initiative to publicly disclose provider performance on selected quality measures. This is done for Medicare Advantage plans, nursing homes, dialysis facilities, and home health agencies through postings to the CMS web site and other mechanisms of public reporting. Information on quality performance is intended to help consumers choose providers and plans, and encourages providers and plans to improve care for beneficiaries. The QIO initiatives and the public reporting tools have been found to be effective ways of improving quality, but their capacity for oversight is limited. For instance, when hospitals or physicians are found to provide poor quality care, the main penalty available is exclusion from the Medicare program, leaving little room for intermediate remedies for less serious offenses.

Historically, other activities to oversee the quality of care include limited utilization review, conditions of participation, and certification of providers. For example, CMS has its own process of certifying hospitals. In addition, it accepts certification of hospitals by the Joint Commission on Accreditation of Healthcare Organizations in lieu of its own hospital certification process. This is referred to as "deemed status." Other providers have also sought deemed status if they meet accreditation standards established by their provider organizations.

CMS also funds state counseling offices to offer information on services, appeals rights, and other basic questions from beneficiaries. These offices provide substantially more information than the "1-800-Medicare" number that also serves beneficiaries. The MMA modestly increased funding for these activities. In addition, the Medicare Ombudsman will pull together information and complaints from beneficiaries. This will be particularly important as the new drug benefit gets underway.

Funding for research has always been part of CMS's responsibilities as well. CMS has broadened its interests to improve data, develop new measures for analysis, and spend additional funds on activities, such as effectiveness research, that may influence both the quality and cost of Medicare. As choices in the Medicare program have expanded, more emphasis has been placed on consumer information and education.

Appendix B

DIFFERENCES IN ESTIMATES OF POVERTY FOR MEDICARE BENEFICIARIES

Different estimates of the number of persons in poverty or near poverty based on income can be obtained from alternative data sources and from differing ways of measuring poverty and income. These estimates affect the number of Medicare beneficiaries assumed to be eligible for a benefit such as the new low-income subsidies for the drug benefit and its perceived generosity in meeting the needs of low-income persons. This appendix attempts to shed some light on why poverty estimates vary so substantially.

SOURCES OF DIFFERENCES

Most of the differences in poverty shares can be explained by four factors:

- The specific definition of poverty used—that is, census thresholds versus Department of Health and Human Services (HHS) guidelines;
- The definition of the unit of measurement;

- The specific survey and the quality of income reporting of data collected;
- The inclusiveness of the population being measured.[1]

Poverty Definitions

Two major sets of poverty measures are commonly used. Molly Orshansky developed the first of these, the census poverty threshold numbers, from a simple formula based on differences in food consumption across families of different size. This measure created the relative differences that are still used today to distinguish across both family size and, for singles and couples, between elderly and younger families. Since this measure has existed since the 1960s and is used by the Census in reporting statistics on poverty, it is the most commonly known and applied measure. Reports each year on whether poverty has increased or decreased, for example, use census data and the census poverty threshold measure. Table B.1 indicates the thresholds for 2004.[2]

The other major alternative measure is the poverty guidelines of the HHS. These guidelines were developed to determine eligibility for public programs such as Supplemental Security Income. They differ from the census numbers in several important respects. First, and particularly important for the Medicare population, the HHS guidelines make no distinctions by age of the family. As a consequence, the poverty cutoff level is set at a higher income for persons age 65 and over, resulting in a higher number of persons in poverty under this measure. Table B.1 contrasts the two sets of poverty cutoff levels for 2004.

Table B.1. Comparisons of Poverty Guidelines and Thresholds, 2004

HHS threshold	
1 person	$9,310
2 persons	$12,490
Census thresholds	
1 person	
Under 65	$9,827
65 and over	$9,060
2 persons	
Under 65	$12,649
65 and over	$11,418
Ratio of HHS threshold to Census threshold for 65 and over	1.03

Source: Author's calculations based on Current Population Survey, 2001, and Medicare Current Beneficiary Survey, 2000.
Note: HHS = Department of Health and Human Services

The Unit of Analysis for Calculating Poverty

Another key issue in estimating poverty is the definition of the family unit whose resources are included in the estimate. For example, if all related persons in a household are included in calculating poverty (the Census approach), the resources of an elderly parent living with her adult child's family would be judged as being in poverty, depending on the resources of this "extended" family, adjusted for family size. However, eligibility for programs is often based on a more narrow definition of resources. The elderly parent's income can be reported separately; indeed, that is more likely to be the income used for determining eligibility for most benefit programs. The Medicare low-income protections, for example, are established on the basis of the individual or couple's income only.

In practice, this has a very large impact on eligibility numbers since many who reside in larger family units do so in order to share scarce resources. The support can go in either direction: sometimes the older family members with the greater resources aid adult children who may have difficulty finding a job or who may have recently been divorced, for example. More commonly, the support flows from the younger family members to a parent or grandparent. As described below, using only the individual's or couple's income increases the number of older persons eligible for assistance.

Differences in Surveys and Data Collection

Since databases are often developed for different purposes and the populations included or excluded can vary substantially, it is necessary to look closely at these differences. This section focuses on comparisons between two databases: the Medicare Current Beneficiary Survey (MCBS), which has the most complete data on use of health care services for the Medicare population, and the Current Population Survey (CPS), which is often viewed as one of the more reliable databases for income and poverty measures.[3]

Constraints on survey length and complexity often dictate that some variables are not measured as well as others. For example, the March CPS is designed to capture carefully the annual income from the year before for American families. Its questions focus on income by source in great detail; this allows the components to be summed, resulting in a smaller chance for underreporting than with the MCBS, which basically asks about annual income in aggregate. Further, the CPS captures income of each family and household member, picking up the income of all family members, such as those in situations where older persons live with younger family members. Again, this provides a very rich database and allows income to be divided into a number of groupings by alternative definitions of family.

The MCBS, by contrast, devotes little time to the income questions since its major focus is on obtaining detailed information about use of health care services, health status, and costs of health care. The MCBS focuses on one person at a time since the Medicare program is individually based. It does capture income for the spouse of the survey respondent, but not for other family members. This can be a disadvantage in measuring all the resources that an individual might have at hand; for example, if she or he is living with other relatives to stretch scarce resources, the survey would not capture these additional resources. Nonetheless, for purposes of eligibility for services that have an income-tested component, only the individual's or married couple's income is relevant. It also likely affects recall; the MCBS is generally acknowledged to have problems with income underreporting.

The Population Covered

Surveys also differ in terms of who is included. The MCBS contains all Medicare beneficiaries, including those in institutions. Institutionalized individuals make up about 5 percent of the Medicare population and their heavy use of Medicare services make them an essential group for study. However, since the institutionalized population is difficult to interview and study, many other surveys, including the CPS, do not include this population. Further, the CPS does not focus on obtaining accurate reporting of Medicare eligibility, so it likely misses a number of younger disability beneficiaries.

How the Numbers Differ in Practice

All of the factors described above help to explain why such large differences in poverty estimates can occur. For example, in published numbers from the 1996 MCBS, the Health Care Financing Administration (HCFA) reported 8.1 million noninstitutionalized beneficiaries with incomes below the Census poverty thresholds (Poisal and Chulis 2000). In contrast, using the standard CPS measure, there were 4.6 million noninstitutionalized Medicare beneficiaries with incomes below the poverty level that year. When translated into shares of the noninstitutionalized population, the respective percentages are 21.8 and 13.0 percent. In this case, the definition of poverty was the same, with the differences being family composition and survey measurement issues. And in 2000, differences remained, although their magnitude declined. In this case, the percentage of noninstitutionalized Medicare beneficiaries measured as poor by the MCBS using HHS guidelines was 17.1 percent, compared with 12.2 percent under the published CPS measure based on census guidelines. And if the institutionalized were included in the MCBS numbers, the share in poverty would have been 18.2 percent.

It is possible to largely reconcile these figures based on the four adjustments described previously. As noted, the two surveys commonly used to estimate poverty for Medicare beneficiaries each have components that do not overlap. Table B.2 demonstrates how to bring the estimates closer together.

The rows in table B.2 are as comparable as possible in terms of the four factors described above. The adjustment that has the largest impact is the change in the unit from which income is derived. Excluding income from other family members substantially increases the share of persons deemed to be in poverty.

Differences between the two surveys may explain the discrepancies that remain and that cannot be corrected for. The MCBS is based on administrative data on enrollment; the CPS uses self-reporting of eligibility. Beneficiaries are often confused about whether they are covered by Medicare or Medicaid, for example. And some respondents usually fail to report participation in any government program. For example, the CPS likely undercounts persons with disabilities receiving Medicare. Further, the MCBS captures persons who died in the 2000 reporting year. This totals over 300,000 persons. The CPS, on the other hand, captures information on people alive in March 2001 and then asks about 2000 information.

Table B.2. Poverty Estimates from Different Surveys, Poverty Definitions, and Family Units, 2000

	Survey used	
	CPS (%)	MCBS (%)
Census thresholds		
Total family	12.2	n.a.
Couple or individual only	16.4	n.a.
HHS guidelines		
Couple or individual only	17.0	17.1

Source: Author's calculations based on Current Population Survey, 2001, and Medicare Current Beneficiary Survey, 2000.

Notes: CPS = Current Population Survey; MCBS = Medicare Current Beneficiary Survey; HHS = Department of Health and Human Services; n.a. = not applicable.

CONCLUSION

There ultimately is no "right" answer concerning the exact number of individuals with incomes below the poverty level. Both surveys, both poverty measures, and various family definitions can be appropriate at different times. The various adjustments described in this appendix help explain why the two surveys have different results. Overall, CPS probably better captures the share of persons living in poverty, although the MCBS includes populations such as decedents and institutionalized persons who would also receive income-related benefits.

NOTES

Chapter 1. The Beneficiary's Perspective

1. All enrollees in Part C are also liable for this Part B premium and may be charged an additional premium for added services as well.

2. Another group that receives employer coverage are those still in the labor force or whose spouse is still working. When these beneficiaries have employer coverage, Medicare becomes the secondary payer (see appendix A).

3. Some individuals maintain plans that they held prior to standardization and other beneficiaries live in states that specify variations on the standardized plans.

4. For a more detailed discussion of the complicated Medicaid program, see Holahan, Wiel, and Wiener 2003.

5. That is, "risk selection" means that plans are paid for patients with average costs, but they have attracted enrollees who are less expensive to serve on average (GAO 2000).

6. In addition to the information provided here, appendix B raises some measurement issues that have complicated discussions over both the absolute and relative economic status of older beneficiaries.

7. Median income captures the income of an individual at the 50th percentile. This is often expressed as the income of a "typical" individual.

8. A family may be as small as two people, such as just the disabled individual and spouse. Also, the category of "family head or spouse" includes heads and spouses of subfamilies within a larger household. These subfamilies tend to be poorer than families with only one nuclear family in the household.

9. The distinction between acute care and long-term care is never absolute. Acute care refers to services, particularly in short-stay hospitals and for physician care, that are used to treat a particular medical condition. Long-term care usually refers to supportive services for persons with chronic disabling

conditions. The numbers described in this volume on out-of-pocket costs include some long term care services offered in the community but none of the costs of institutional care aside from skilled nursing facility payments.

Chapter 2. Medicare in the "Big Picture"

1. U.S. Department of Labor, Bureau of Labor Statistics, "Most Requested Statistics, Consumer Price Index," Internet communication.

2. It should be noted that price increases in medical care, like other parts of the CPI, may be overstated (Huskamp and Newhouse 1994). Quality improvements and price discounting are not well captured by this measure. But in comparative terms, the differences are still dramatic.

3. Although there is also a Part B Trust Fund, it serves a much different purpose and is intentionally kept at a small positive level.

4. Unlike the Social Security Trust Fund to which additional revenues were added in 1983 to "pre-fund" some of its benefits, Medicare's Part A Trust Fund was not adjusted to take on such a role. Instead, improvements in projections of solvency have largely arisen from changes on the spending side.

5. When Medicare begins to redeem its securities (because benefit costs begin to exceed trust fund receipts), the burdens of meeting these obligations will fall on citizens. At that point, general revenue taxes can be raised, spending on other services can be reduced, or the Treasury can redeem Medicare's securities by issuing new debt to the public. If the debt owed to the public were reduced through 2015 using Medicare's surpluses, then it would be easier to increase borrowing at a later time, helping to finance extra contributions to Medicare. But using the surplus to finance current spending (even on Part B) or to cut other taxes eliminates this advantage.

6. Formal analyses of federal spending by both the Congressional Budget Office and by the Office of Management and Budget in the administrative branch use current law for any projections. Yet the alternative these two agencies suggest violate that long-standing principle.

7. We use 2035 since it will capture much of the dramatic growth in Medicare spending. The uncertainty of estimates beyond 2035 is such that it may be very misleading to project until 2075 as is required of the Trustees Report. The 2075 figure is not much lower, however, settling at 2.0.

8. Indeed, this has been the justification over the years for increasing Social Security benefit generosity and adding Medicare to the system. In that way, the higher standards of living Americans have enjoyed since the end of World War II were shared with retirees.

9. The figure used here is based on the intermediate projections from the 2002 Trustees Report, which assumes a 1.1 percent real growth in per-worker wages each year. Over the past 50 years, productivity has been higher than this amount, averaging over 1.5 percent per year. The calculations for this measure are discussed in more detail in Moon and Storeygard (2002).

10. This trend has been in place since 1975 as well, with Medicare burdens growing but not by enough to slow the growth in per-worker resources by very much. In addition, the results would be similar if we were to add Social Security to this calculation.

Chapter 3. How Medicare Has Changed: Coverage and Benefit Payments

1. In 1950, the Old Age Assistance program also established a system of vendor payments to providers of health care for the elderly, but with even more limited federal dollars.

2. Some states continued their MAA programs after 1965, as allowed by law, in lieu of Medicaid for the elderly. MAA was eliminated in 1969.

3. Medicaid is, like MAA, a joint federal and state program in which the federal government sets some rules and provides matching monies to states. The states must provide benefits to those eligible for cash assistance. Certain benefits are federally mandated. Beyond that, the states may choose to cover additional services and additional beneficiaries under the medically needy provision. Medicaid is available to persons of all ages. Over time, its importance for the elderly has been primarily for long-term care services not covered by Medicare and as a supplemental program filling Medicare's gaps for those with very low incomes.

4. Senator Long also argued for means-tested cost sharing. Although that provision was not included in the legislation, it is interesting that the issues Long raised began to resurface in the late 1980s as a potential direction for change in Medicare.

5. Indeed, the system was so successful that critics both then and later pointed to the danger of the increasing costs of health care—a criticism that proved well founded. Perhaps the AMA got the last laugh after all. A *New York Times* article on August 19, 1966, indicated that physicians' prices for the elderly rose by 300 percent on the introduction of Medicare.

6. This ratio is likely to decline even faster now for those who pay at the maximum since the cap on earnings subject to the tax increased in 1991.

7. The 1972 amendments also allowed individuals over age 65 to buy into Part A if they were not otherwise eligible and established a few minor expansions of services. These amendments also raised the Part B deductible from $50 to $60 and, in what would become an important change over time, tied premium increases in Part B to the newly added Social Security cost of living adjustment (COLA) (U.S. Social Security Administration 1991).

8. Younger workers have lesser requirements, and persons in other categories such as disabled adult children must meet other standards.

9. This issue has again been raised in the context of eligibility for the AIDS population. Many AIDS victims will die before becoming eligible for Medicare through the traditional disability program. Advocates for AIDS patients thus urge that, as is now the case for ESRD, there should be no waiting period.

10. This expansion was less generous than for ESRD, which has no work eligibility requirements.

11. Interestingly, efforts to create universal coverage in the 1990s avoided building on the Medicare model. But in 2003, Senator Ted Kennedy made a speech calling for Medicare for all.

12. Except for the period when disability determinations were consciously held down, growth in the number of disability beneficiaries has not been well understood.

13. Legislation in 1997 folded this commission into a broader Medicare Payment Assessment Commission (MedPAC).

14. Another number commonly cited is $115.1 billion, which is a net savings figure after accounting for increased Medicaid expenditures as a result of Medicare changes.

15. See p. H6177 of the July 29, 1997, *Congressional Record*. A defined contribution approach—where Medicare only guarantees a fixed dollar contribution and not benefits—would represent a major change in the nature of the entitlement. Because the new private fee-for-service and medical savings account options may charge beneficiaries additional premiums for expanded services and are not required to offer a basic option, implicitly, they are no longer guaranteeing a set benefit and hence constitute a defined contribution approach.

16. The BBA also reduced payments to certain managed care plans by $4 billion over five years by "carving out" payments for medical education that had effectively been built into the capitated rate. Hospitals entitled to these payments had argued that HMOs failed to pass on such payments to them and instead were simply reaping a windfall from the calculation of the monthly payment rate.

Chapter 4. How Medicare Has Changed: Benefits

1. Kidney dialysis treatments were added in 1972 when end stage renal disease patients were made eligible, as discussed in chapter 3.

2. The approach recognized that a $2,000 cap on spending was too high to protect the poor from "unaffordable" health care costs, and since the change was to be added through Medicaid, it would not seem to be "means testing" the benefits. These benefits, later expanded and renamed the Medicare Savings Program, are still largely in place. The spousal impoverishment provisions raised the amount of income and assets a spouse could keep when the husband or wife received Medicaid support for nursing home expenses, thus increasing the number of people eligible for Medicaid.

3. This eliminated the concept of a spell of illness which allowed multiple deductibles to be charged in any given year.

4. The exception to this is that state pharmaceutical benefit programs will be allowed to fill in the gaps for people eligible for these benefits. At present, only four states have plans that provide benefits to substantial numbers of people with incomes above 150 percent of the federal poverty level. In addition, there is no penalty on employer-subsidized plans that are more comprehensive than the new benefit package. In fact, as long as the package provides coverage at least at the level of the basic plan, employers will qualify for a subsidy toward the costs of that benefit.

5. These figures represent the spending distribution for all beneficiaries, and thus the distribution for those who participate in the program and who do not have low-income subsidies may vary.

6. Institutionalized individuals face no cost-sharing requirements, and those with incomes below 100 percent of the poverty level who are dually eligible have slightly lower cost-sharing requirements.

7. Some of these individuals, however, might be enrolled in state-only pharmaceutical benefit plans. This estimate is contained in a Congressional Budget Office letter to Senator Don Nickles, November 20, 2003.

8. This calculation assumes an annual income in 2006 of $15,400 and includes the premium and cost-sharing required.

9. That is, Medicare makes direct payments to hospitals for these expenses and that amount is averaged over all beneficiaries as a Medicare cost. But, since private plans do not pay such subsidies to hospitals, they effectively receive an overpayment. These overpayments were taken out of payments to private plans in the Balanced Budget Act of 1997, but the current legislation would restore these amounts.

10. Comments by Robert Reischauer and Jeff Lemieux at Alliance for Health Reform meeting, 2003.

11. Patients relying on multiple doctors or who are in the middle of treatments are less likely to want to face the disruption of changing plans, for example.

Chapter 5. Are Private Plans the Answer for Medicare?

1. Often viewed as a logical next step would be to shift Medicare's commitment from that of a defined benefit to a defined contribution approach, allowing even more federal control over the costs of Medicare. This approach, however, would simply shift costs onto beneficiaries. This option will thus be considered in chapter 7.

2. This decline was mitigated by the emergence of private fee-for-service plans, which modestly increased access to private plans over the period.

Chapter 6. How Could the Benefit Structure Be Improved?

1. The Medicare Catastrophic Coverage Act of 1988 would certainly count if it had not been repealed just a year later.

2. The estimated actuarial value of the new drug benefit, if implemented in 2004, would be $735 per capita, so the net costs above basic Medicare plus drug coverage would be $592 for Medicare Extra.

3. The Congressional Budget Office has always indicated that there would be savings if Medigap were required to be less comprehensive, thus leaving beneficiaries to face more cost sharing than currently happens under the combination of traditional Medicare and Medigap (see CBO 2005). Beneficiaries would face greater cost sharing if people received a more generous benefit through Medicare and stopped purchasing Medigap.

4. A number of other adjustments would be needed to change cost sharing, however, since Parts A and B are now separate programs. And contrary to what some analysts have claimed, many insurance plans—including those found in the Federal Employees Health Benefits Program, which is often cited as a model for Medicare—have two or more deductibles.

5. Note, however, that the options shown here also limit the number of Part A deductibles to just one per year.

Chapter 7. Who Should Pay?

1. To keep the analysis simple, payments from Medicaid and employers have been omitted, focusing only on Medicare and individual contributions.

2. This calculation ignores the costs of long-term care, which fall even more heavily on individuals.

3. For the moment, this calculation ignores Part D, which has just started. Once it is added, the share of Medicare A, B, and D paid by premiums will rise.

4. The issue of timing of a tax increase and how trust fund balances will be treated is discussed at the end of this chapter.

5. The analysis focuses on the VAT rather than the retail sales tax because there is greater worldwide experience with a national VAT. Also, some have raised concerns about the problems of compliance with a national retail sales tax. However, because the two forms of tax are essentially equivalent (assuming they could be equally well administered), the revenue and incidence effects of the two forms of consumption tax would be quite similar.

Chapter 8. How Should Medicare Change?

1. An alternative to a stop-loss approach would be to eliminate hospital coinsurance and multiple deductibles in any given year. This would not achieve as much protection for beneficiaries, however, since it is the unlimited nature of Part B coinsurance that usually results in high out-of-pocket liabilities.

2. Since most of the estimates of the cost of the drug plans have assumed high levels of participation, making the benefit mandatory should not create a substantial problem for most beneficiaries. Low-income protection limits might need to be raised to ensure affordability of the premium to those earning 150 to 200 percent of the poverty level, for example.

3. These numbers are low because the census poverty estimates do not fully capture all those who could be eligible. These numbers exclude the disabled, and the poverty calculations used differ from the number counted as low income for purposes of program eligibility (see appendix B).

Appendix A. The Mechanics of Medicare

1. Unless otherwise noted, material for this appendix is drawn from several sources that detail the workings of the Medicare program. For more information, see U.S. Congress, Committee on Ways and Means (2000); Commerce Clearing House (2003); Boards of Trustees (2004); U.S. Department of Health and Human Services (2001, 2003); and Medicare Payment Advisory Commission (2003a).

2. In 2000, persons with amyotrophic lateral sclerosis (ALS) were excepted from this two-year "waiting period."

3. Medicare beneficiaries who have even lower incomes qualify for full Medicaid benefits. In addition to covering these beneficiaries' Medicare premiums, deductibles, and coinsurance, Medicaid provides coverage for non-Medicare benefits, such as prescription drugs and extended long-term care.

4. Inpatient psychiatric services are limited to 190 days over a patient's lifetime.

5. For many years, home health care was largely provided under Part A. It was shifted to Part B in 1998. This shift, phased in over time, had two major effects: (1) it reduced Part A spending and hence extended the date of exhaustion of the Part A trust fund, and (2) it increased beneficiary burdens through an increase in the Part B premium.

6. In the 1980s, elderly advocates criticized the dual, and essentially conflicting, requirements of intermittency and confinement to the home as a catch-22 that precluded eligibility for many Medicare enrollees. Easing intermittency guidelines in the 1990s lessened this problem and expanded use of this benefit.

7. Medicare Payment Advisory Commission, "Improving the Medicare + Choice Program: Recommendations of MedPAC." Testimony before the U.S. Senate Committee on Finance, April 3, 2001.

8. Coinsurance is a charge assessed against the user of a service that is defined as a percentage of the cost of that care. The term cost sharing normally refers to coinsurance and deductibles—the costs of care that beneficiaries are required to "share." Technically, this is not coinsurance—although it is the term that Medicare uses—since it is not tied to the cost of SNF care, but, rather, to the cost of hospital services.

9. Even after the recent requirement that physicians file claims for their patients, they can ask for payment directly from the beneficiary rather than being paid by Medicare.

10. These periodic interim payments (PIPs) were originally established to smooth the cash flow for hospitals. In the 1980s, they became a convenient, albeit bogus, device to achieve Medicare "savings." By delaying the payment from one fiscal year to the next, Medicare appears to have been cut.

Appendix B. Differences in Estimates of Poverty for Medicare Beneficiaries

1. Two other issues not pursued here are the question of what types of income are excluded from eligibility determination and how asset tests can further reduce the number of eligibles.

2. Note also, however, that the Census also publishes alternative poverty measures, some of which are directly relevant here because they capture health care costs by individuals. In this case, the poverty rates for persons age 65 and older are much higher.

3. Each database also has its detractors. For example, the CPS is sometimes criticized for underreporting certain types of income, meaning that poverty rates might be even lower than it finds. And detractors of the MCBS point out its problems in underreporting drug spending. Nonetheless, these are likely the two most important data sources for comparisons of poverty rates for the Medicare population.

REFERENCES

Alexcih, Lisa M. B., Steven Lutzky, Purvi Sevak, and Gary Claxton. 1997. *Key Issues Affecting Accessibility to Medigap Insurance*. New York: The Commonwealth Fund.

American Academy of Actuaries. 2002. "Understanding Defined Contribution Health Plans." Issue Brief. Washington, DC: American Academy of Actuaries.

American Hospital Association. 1995. *Hospital Statistics*. Chicago: American Hospital Association.

Andersen, Ronald, Joanna Lion, and Odin W. Anderson. 1976. *Two Decades of Health Services: Social Survey Trends in Use and Expenditure*. Cambridge, MA: Ballinger Publishing Company.

Andersen, Ronald, Joanna Kravits, Odin W. Anderson, and Joan Daley. 1973. *Expenditures for Personal Health Services: National Hands and Variations, 1953–1970*. Washington, DC: U.S. Department of Health, Education, and Welfare.

Angeles, January, and Marilyn Moon. Forthcoming. "Improving Medicare Coverage: Next Steps in Fee for Service." Washington, DC: authors.

Antos, Joseph., and Roland E. King. 2003. *Comparing Medicare and Private-Sector Spending Growth: Recent Study Does Not Account for Important Private-Sector Changes*. Washington, DC: Pharmaceutical Research and Manufacturers of America.

Barents Group. 1999. *A Profile of QMB-Eligible and SLMB-Eligible Medicare Beneficiaries*. Baltimore, MD: Health Care Financing Administration.

Biles, Brian, L. Nicholas, and Barbara S. Cooper. 2004. "The Cost of Privatization: Extra Payments to Medicare Advantage Plans—2005 Update." Washington, DC: The Commonwealth Fund.

Board of Trustees. 1981. *1981 Annual Report of the Board of Trustees of the Federal Hospital Insurance Trust Fund*. Washington, DC: U.S. Government Printing Office.

———. 1996. *1996 Annual Report of the Board of Trustees of the Federal Hospital Insurance Trust Fund.* Washington, DC: U.S. Government Printing Office.

———. 1997. *1997 Annual Report of the Board of Trustees of the Federal Hospital Insurance Trust Fund.* Washington, DC: U.S. Government Printing Office.

———. 1998. *1998 Annual Report of the Board of Trustees of the Federal Hospital Insurance Trust Fund.* Washington, DC: U.S. Government Printing Office.

———. 2000. *2000 Annual Report of the Board of Trustees of the Federal Hospital Insurance Trust Fund.* Washington, DC: U.S. Government Printing Office.

Boards of Trustees. 2004. *2004 Annual Report of the Boards of Trustees of the Federal Hospital Insurance and Federal Supplementary Medical Insurance Trust Funds.* Washington, DC: U.S. Government Printing Office.

———. 2005. *2005 Annual Report of the Boards of Trustees of the Federal Hospital Insurance and Federal Supplementary Medical Insurance Trust Funds.* Washington, DC: U.S. Government Printing Office.

Boccuti, Cristina, and Marilyn Moon. 2003. "Comparing Medicare and Private Insurance: Growth Rates in Spending over Three Decades." *Health Affairs* 22:230–37.

Boccuti, Cristina, Marilyn Moon, and Krista Dowling. 2003. "Chronic Conditions and Disabilities: Trends and Issues for Private Drug Plans." Issue Brief. New York: The Commonwealth Fund.

Brown, Randall, Dolores G. Clement, Jerrold W. Hill, Sheldon Retchin, and Jeanette Bergeron. 1993. "Do Health Maintenance Organizations Work for Medicare?" *Health Care Financing Review* 15 (Fall): 7–23.

Buchmueller, Thomas. 2000. "The Health Plan Choices of Retirees under Managed Competition." *Health Affairs* 35:949–76.

Campion, Frank D. 1984. *AMA and U.S. Health Policy since 1940.* Chicago: Chicago Review Press.

CBO. *See* U.S. Congressional Budget Office.

Centers for Medicare and Medicaid Services. 2003. "Medicare + Choice: Access and Benefits." Conference presentation sponsored by the Agency for Healthcare Research and Quality, April 29.

———. 2004a. *Health Care Financing Review: Annual Statistical Supplement, 2003.* Washington, DC: U.S. Government Printing Office.

———. 2004b. *Medicare Preferred Provider Organization (PPO) Demonstration Fact Sheet.* Washington, DC: U.S. Government Printing Office.

Chollet, Deborah. 2003. "The Medigap Market: Product and Pricing Trends, 1999–2001." *Monitoring Medicare + Choice Operational Insights* 11 (October). Washington, DC: Mathematica Policy Research, Inc.

Christensen, Sandra. 1991. "Did 1980s Legislation Slow Medicare Spending?" *Health Affairs* 10(2): 135–42.

———. 1992. "The Subsidy Provided under Medicare to Current Enrollees." *Journal of Health Politics, Policy, and Law* 17 (Summer): 255–64.

Christensen, Sandra, and Richard Kasten. 1988. "Covering Catastrophic Expenses under Medicare." *Health Affairs* 7 (Winter): 79–93.

Christianson, Jon, Stephen Parente, and Ruth Taylor. 2002. "Defined-Contribution Health Insurance Products: Development and Prospects." *Health Affairs* 21(1): 49–64.

Clark, Robert L., Richard V. Burkhauser, Marilyn Moon, Joseph F. Quinn, and Timothy M. Smeeding. 2004. *The Economics of an Aging Society.* Melbourne, Australia: Blackwell Publishing Ltd.

References ■ 217

CMS. *See* Centers for Medicare and Medicaid Services.
Collins, Sara, Karen Davis, Cathy Schoen, Michelle Doty, Sabrina How, and Alyssa Holmgren. 2005. *Will You Still Need Me? The Health and Financial Security of Older Americans: Findings from the Commonwealth Fund Survey of Older Adults.* New York: The Commonwealth Fund.
Commerce Clearing House. 2003. *2003 Medicare Explained.* Chicago: Commerce Clearing House, Inc.
Congressional Research Service. 1989. "Health Insurance and the Uninsured: Background Data and Analysis." Washington, DC: U.S. Senate Committee on Education and Labor.
Connolly, Ceci. 2006. "HHS Works to Fix Drug Plan Woes." *Washington Post,* January 18, p. A3.
Council of Economic Advisors. 1964. "Economic Report of the President." Washington, DC: U.S. Government Printing Office.
Cutler, David. 2004. *Your Money or Your Life: Strong Medicine for America's Health Care System.* New York: Oxford University Press.
Dale, Stacy B., and James M. Verdier. 2003. *Elimination of Medicare's Waiting Period for Seriously Disabled Adults: Impact on Coverage and Costs.* New York: The Commonwealth Fund.
Davis, Karen, and Cathy Schoen. 1978. *Health and the War on Poverty: A Ten-Year Appraisal.* Washington, DC: Brookings Institution Press.
Davis, Karen, Cathy Schoen, Melissa Doty, and Katie Tenney. 2002. "Medicare Versus Private Insurance: Rhetoric and Reality." *Health Affairs* web exclusive. http://www.healthaffairs.org.
Davis, Karen, Marilyn Moon, Barbara Cooper, and Cathy Schoen. 2005. "Medicare Extra: A Comprehensive Benefit Option for Medicare Beneficiaries." *Health Affairs* web exclusive, October 4. http://www.healthaffairs.org.
Derthick, Martha. 1979. *Policymaking for Social Security.* Washington, DC: Brookings Institution Press.
Doty, Pamela, Korbin Liu, and Joshua Wiener. 1985. "An Overview of Long-Term Care." *Health Care Financing Review* 5 (Spring): 69–78.
Dyckman, Zachary, and Pamela Hess. 2002. *Survey of Health Plans Concerning Physician Fees and Payment Methodology.* Washington, DC: Medicare Payment Advisory Commission.
Feder, Judith. 1977. *Medicare: The Politics of Federal Hospital Insurance.* Lexington, MA: DC Health and Company.
Feder, Judith, John Holahan, Randall R. Bovbjerg, and Jack Hadley. 1982. "Health." In *The Reagan Experiment,* edited by John L. Palmer and Isabel V. Sawhill (271–306). Washington, DC: Urban Institute Press.
Federal Interagency Forum on Aging-Related Statistics. 2004. *Older Americans 2004: Key Indicators of Well-Being.* Washington, DC: U.S. Government Printing Office.
Fox, Peter D., R. E. Snyder, and Thomas Rice. 2003. "Medigap Reform Legislation of 1990: A 10-year Review." *Health Care Financing Review* 24:121–37.
Freudenheim, Milt. 2004. "Cost of Insuring Workers' Health Increases 11.2%." *New York Times,* September 10, p. C1.
GAO. *See* U.S. Government Accountability Office *and* U.S. General Accounting Office.
Gluck, Michael, and Marilyn Moon. 2000. *Financing Medicare's Future: Final Report of the Study Panel on Medicare's Long Term Care Financing.* Washington, DC: National Academy of Social Insurance.

Gold, Marsha, and Lori Achman. 2003. "Average Out-of-Pocket Health Care Costs for Medicare + Choice Enrollees Increase 10 Percent in 2003." New York: Commonwealth Fund.

Gold, Marsha, and Lindsay Harris. 2005. "Profile and Analysis of the 26 Medicare Advantage Regions." Menlo Park, CA: Henry J. Kaiser Family Foundation.

Grad, Susan. 1989. "Income and Assets of Social Security Beneficiaries by Type of Benefit." *Social Security Bulletin* 52:2–10.

———. 2003. *Income of the Aged Chartbook.* Washington, DC: Social Security Administration.

HCFA. *See* Health Care Financing Administration.

Health Care Financing Administration. 1995. "Health Care Financing Review Medicare and Medicaid Statistical Supplement, 1995." Baltimore, MD: U.S. Department of Health and Human Services.

Height, Dorothy I. 1996. "Thirty Years of Medicare: A Personal Reflection on Medicare's Impact on Black Americans." *Health Care Financing Review* 18(2): 87–90.

Henry J. Kaiser Family Foundation. 2000. *Faces of Medicare.* Washington, DC: Henry J. Kaiser Family Foundation.

Henry J. Kaiser Family Foundation and Health Research and Educational Trust. 2004. *Employer Health Benefits: 2004 Annual Survey.* Menlo Park, CA, and Chicago: Henry J. Kaiser Family Foundation and Health Research and Educational Trust.

Henry J. Kaiser Family Foundation and Hewitt Associates LLC. 2004. *Current Trends and Future Outlook for Retiree Health Benefits: Findings from the Kaiser/Hewitt 2004 Survey on Retiree Health Benefits.* Menlo Park, CA, and Lincolnshire, IL: Henry J. Kaiser Family Foundation and Hewitt Associates LLC.

Hewitt Associates LLC. 2000. *The Implications of Medicare Prescription Drug Proposals for Employers and Retirees.* Menlo Park, CA: Henry J. Kaiser Family Foundation.

Holahan, John, and Mary Beth Pohl. 2003. "Leaders and Laggards in State Coverage Expansions." *Federalism and Health Policy* 179:186–91.

Holahan, John, Alan Weil, and Joshua Wiener, eds. 2003. *Federalism and Health Policy.* Washington, DC: Urban Institute Press.

Holtz-Eakin, Douglas. 2004. "Estimating the Cost of the Medicare Modernization Act." Testimony before the U.S. Congress, Committee on Ways and Means, March 24. Washington, DC: Congressional Budget Office.

Hsiao, William C., Peter Braun, Edmund Becker, Nancyanne Causino, Nathan Couch, Margaret DeNicola, Daniel Dunn, Nancy Kelly, Thomas Ketcham, Arthur Sobol, Diana Verrilli, and Douwe Yntema. 1988. *A National Study of Resource-Based Relative Value Scales for Physician Services.* Cambridge, MA: Harvard University.

Huskamp, Haiden, and Joseph Newhouse. 1994. "Is Health Spending Slowing Down?" *Health Affairs* 13 (Winter): 32–38.

Kaiser Family Foundation. *See* Henry J. Kaiser Family Foundation.

Kenney, Genevieve. 1991. "Understanding the Effects of the PPS on Medicare Home Health Use." *Inquiry* 28:129–39.

Kenney, Genevieve, and Marilyn Moon. 1995. *Medicare Subacute Care Services and Enrollee Characteristics.* Washington, DC: The Urban Institute.

Kozak, Lola J., Eileen McCarthy, and Robert Pokras. 1999. "Changing Patterns of Surgical Care in the United States, 1980–1995." *Health Care Financing Review* 21:31–49.

Langwell, Kathryn, and James Hadley. 1989. "Evaluation of the Medicare Competition Demonstrations." *Health Care Financing Review* 11 (Winter): 65–79.

Leader, Shelah, and Marilyn Moon. 1989. "Medicare Trends in Ambulatory Surgery." *Health Affairs* (Spring): 158–70.

Lesser, Cynthia S., Paul B. Ginsburg, and Kelly J. Devers. 2003. "The End of an Era: What Became of the 'Managed Care Revolution' in 2001?" *Health Services Research* 38.

Liu, Korbin, and Genevieve Kenney. 1991. *Impact of the Catastrophic Coverage Act and New Coverage Guidelines on the Medicare SNF Benefit.* Washington, DC: The Urban Institute.

Luft, Hal S., and Edward M. Morrison. 1991. "Alternative Delivery Systems." In *Health Services Research: Key to Health Policy,* edited by E. Ginzberg (195–233). Cambridge, MA: Harvard University Press.

Marmor, Theodore R. 1970. *The Politics of Medicare.* Chicago: Aldine Publishing Co.

Maxwell, Stephanie, Marilyn Moon, and Misha Segal. 2001. *Growth in Medicare and Out-of-Pocket Spending: Impact on Vulnerable Beneficiaries.* New York: The Commonwealth Fund.

Medicare Payment Advisory Commission. 1998. *A Data Book: Health Care Spending and the Medicare Program.* Washington, DC: MedPAC.

———. 2000. *Report to Congress: Medicare Payment Policy.* Washington, DC: MedPAC.

———. 2001. *Report to Congress: Medicare Payment Policy.* Washington, DC: MedPAC.

———. 2002. *Report to Congress: Assessing Medicare Benefits.* Washington, DC: MedPAC.

———. 2003a. *A Data Book: Healthcare Spending and the Medicare Program.* Washington, DC: MedPAC.

———. 2003b. *Report to Congress: Medicare Payment Policy 153.* Washington, DC: MedPAC.

———. 2004a. *Report to Congress: New Approaches in Medicare.* Washington, DC: MedPAC.

———. 2004b. *Report to Congress: Medicare Payment Policy 211.* Washington, DC: MedPAC.

———. 2005. *A Data Book: Healthcare Spending and the Medicare Program.* Washington, DC: MedPAC.

Medicare Rights Center. 2002. "An Investigative Report on Medicare Savings Programs in New York City: Local and State Involvement in Federal Programs Impedes Access for People with Low Incomes." http://www.medicarerights.org.

MedPAC. See Medicare Payment Advisory Commission.

Metlife Mature Market Institute. 2004. *2004 Metlife Mature Market Institute Survey Report* Hartford, CT: Metlife.

Moon, Marilyn. 1996. *Medicare Now and in the Future,* 2nd ed. Washington, DC: Urban Institute Press.

————. 1999. "Beneath the Averages: An Analysis of Medicare and Private Expenditures." Menlo Park, CA: The Henry J. Kaiser Family Foundation, 1999.

Moon, Marilyn, and Cristina Boccuti. 2002. "Location, Location, Location: Geographic Spending Issues and Medicare Policy." Health Policy Brief no. 2. Washington, DC: The Urban Institute.

Moon, Marilyn, and Barbara Gage. 1997. "Key Medicare Provisions in the Balanced Budget Act of 1997." *Public Policy and Aging Report* Fall: 8.

Moon, Marilyn, and Matthew Storeygard. 2001. "One Third at Risk: The Special Circumstances of Medicare Beneficiaries with Health Problems." New York: The Commonwealth Fund.

————. 2002. *Solvency or Affordability? Ways to Measure Medicare's Financial Health.* Washington, DC: The Henry J. Kaiser Family Foundation.

Moon, Marilyn, Robert Freidland, and Lee Shirey. 2002. *Medicare Beneficiaries and Their Assets: Implications for Low-Income Programs.* Menlo Park, CA: Henry J. Kaiser Family Foundation.

Moon, Marilyn, Barbara Gage, and Allison Evans. 1997. *An Examination of Key Medicare Provisions in the Balanced Budget Act of 1997.* Washington, DC: The Commonwealth Fund.

Moon, Marilyn, Misha Segal, and Randall Weiss. 2000/2001. "A Moving Target: Financing Medicare for the Future." *Inquiry* 37(4): 338–47.

Myers, Robert J. 1970. *Medicare.* Homewood, IL: Richard D. Irwin.

National Center for Health Statistics. 1991. *Health, United States, 1990.* Hyattsville, MD: Public Health Service.

————. 1996. *Health, United States, 1995.* Hyattsville, MD: Public Health Service.

————. 2002. *Health, United States, 2002, with Chartbook on Trends in the Health of Americans.* Washington, DC: U.S. Government Printing Office.

————. 2003. *Health, United States, 2003, with Chartbook on Trends in the Health of Americans.* Hyattsville, MD: National Center for Health Statistics.

National Research Council. 1995. *Measuring Poverty: A New Approach.* Washington, DC: National Academy Press.

NCHS. *See* National Center for Health Statistics.

Nemore, Patricia. 2005. "Medicare Part D: Issues for Dual Eligibles on the Eve of Implementation." Menlo Park, CA: Henry J. Kaiser Family Foundation.

Newhouse, Joseph, Melinda B. Buntin, and John Chapman. 1999. *Risk Adjustment and Medicare.* New York: The Commonwealth Fund.

Newman, Howard N. 1972. "Medicare and Medicaid." *Annals of the American Academy of Political and Social Science* 399 (January): 114–24.

Nichols, Len, and Robert Reischauer. 2000. "Who Really Wants Price Competition in Medicare Managed Care?" *Health Affairs* 19 (September/October): 30–43.

Nichols, Len M., Paul M. Ginsburg, and Robert A. Berenson. 2004. "Are Market Forces Strong Enough to Deliver Efficient Health Care Systems? Confidence Is Waning." *Health Affairs* 23:8–21.

Oberlander, Jonathan. 2003. *The Political Life of Medicare.* Chicago: University of Chicago Press.

Office of Technology Assessment. 1985. *Medicare's Prospective Payment System: Strategies for Evaluating Cost, Quality, and Medical Technology.* Washington, DC: U.S. Government Printing Office.

Pauly, Mark. 2004. "Means-Testing in Medicare." *Health Affairs* web exclusive, December 8. http://www.healthaffairs.org.

Pear, Robert. 2003. "Bush May Link Drug Benefit in Medicare to Private Plans." *New York Times*, January 24.

———. 2005. "Over a Million on Medicare Sign up for New Drug Plan." *New York Times*, December 23, p. A1.

Physician Payment Review Commission. 1987. *Medicare Physician Payment: An Agenda for Reform.* Washington, DC: U.S. Government Printing Office.

Plotnick, Robert, and Felicity Skidmore. 1976. *Progress against Poverty: A Review of the 1964–1974 Decade.* New York: Academic Press.

Poisal, John, and George Chulis. 2000. "Medicare Beneficiaries and Drug Coverage." *Health Affairs* 19 (March/April): 248–56.

Pollitz, Karen, Richard Sorian, and Kathy Thomas. 2001. *How Accessible Is Individual Health Insurance for Consumers in Less-Than-Perfect Health?* Menlo Park, CA: The Henry J. Kaiser Family Foundation.

Poterba, James, and Lawrence Summers. 1985. *Public Policy Implications of Declining Old-Age Mortality.* Cambridge, MA: National Bureau of Economic Research.

PPRC. *See* Physician Payment Review Commission.

Rettig, Richard. 1976. "The Policy Debate on Patient Care Financing for Victims of End-Stage Renal Disease." *Law and Contemporary Problems* 40 (Autumn): 196–230.

———. 1982. "The Federal Government and Social Planning for End-Stage Renal Disease: Past, Present, and Future." *Seminars in Nephrology* 2 (June): 111–33.

Rich, Spencer. 1987. " 'Catastrophic' Bill's Cost Raises New Doubt." *The Washington Post*, September 14.

Scandlen, Greg. 2000. *Defined Contribution Health Insurance.* Dallas: National Center for Policy Analysis.

Shapiro, Isaac, and Joel Friedman. 2004. "Tax Returns: A Comprehensive Assessment of the Bush Administration's Record on Cutting Taxes." Washington, DC: Center on Budget and Policy Priorities. http://www.cbpp.org/4-14-04tax-sum.htm.

Simon, Matt. 1989. "Flimflam: The National Committee and Its Pitch to Seniors." *Union* (April/May): 13–16.

Skidmore, Max J. 1970. *Medicare and the American Rhetoric of Reconciliation.* Tuscaloosa, AL: University of Alabama Press.

Smits, Helen, Judith Feder, and William Scanlon. 1982. "Medicare's Nursing Home Benefit: Variations in Interpretation." *New England Journal of Medicine* 307:855–62.

Social Security Administration. 1991. *Social Security Bulletin, Annual Statistical Supplement.* Washington, DC: U.S. Government Printing Office.

———. 2003. *Annual Statistical Supplement to the Social Security Bulletin.* Washington, DC: Social Security Administration.

Somers, Herman M., and Anne R. Somers. 1967. *Medicare and the Hospitals: Issues and Prospects.* Washington, DC: The Brookings Institution.

Starr, Paul. 1982. *The Social Transformation of American Medicine.* New York: Basic Books.

Stevens, Rosemary A. 1996. "Health Care in the Early 1960s." *Health Care Financing Review* 18(2): 11–22.

Strunk, Bradley, Paul Ginsburg, and Jon Gabel. 2002. "Tracking Health Care Costs: Growth Accelerates Again in 2001." *Health Affairs* web exclusive: w299–w310.

Sulvetta, Margaret. 1992. "Achieving Cost Control in the Hospital Outpatient Department." *Health Care Financing Review* (Annual Supplement): 95–106.

Summer, Laura, and Robert Freidland. 2002. *The Role of the Asset Test in Targeting Benefits for Medicare Savings Programs.* Washington, DC: The Commonwealth Fund.

Tang, Paul, and David Lansky. 2005. "The Missing Link: Bridging the Patient-Provider Health Information Gap." *Health Affairs* 24(4): 1290–95.

Torres-Gil, Fernando. 1989. "The Politics of Catastrophic and Long-term Care Coverage." *Journal of Aging and Social Policy* 12:61–86.

U.S. Bureau of the Census. 1991. *Money Income of Households, Families, and Persons in the United States: 1990.* Washington, DC: U.S. Government Printing Office.

———. 1995. *Income, Poverty, and Valuation of Noncash Benefits: 1993.* Washington, DC: U.S. Government Printing Office.

———. 2004. *Income, Poverty, and Health Insurance Coverage in the United States: 2003.* Report no. P60-226. Washington, DC: U.S. Bureau of the Census.

U.S. Congress, Committee on Ways and Means. 1985. *1985 Green Book: Background Material and Data on Programs within the Jurisdiction of the Committee on Ways and Means.* Washington, DC: U.S. Government Printing Office.

———. 1989. *1989 Green Book: Background Material and Data on Programs within the Jurisdiction of the Committee on Ways and Means.* Washington, DC: U.S. Government Printing Office.

———. 1991. *1991 Green Book: Background Material and Data on Programs within the Jurisdiction of the Committee on Ways and Means.* Washington, DC: U.S. Government Printing Office.

———. 1992. *1992 Green Book: Background Material and Data on Programs within the Jurisdiction of the Committee on Ways and Means.* Washington, DC: U.S. Government Printing Office.

———. 1994. *1994 Green Book: Background Material and Data on Programs within the Jurisdiction of the Committee on Ways and Means.* Washington, DC: U.S. Government Printing Office.

———. 2000. *2000 Green Book: Overview of Entitlement Programs.* Washington, DC: U.S. Government Printing Office.

U.S. Congressional Budget Office. 1983. *Changing the Structure of Medicare Benefits: Issues and Options—A CBO Study.* Washington, DC: U.S. Government Printing Office.

———. 1987. *Background Information on Out-of-Pocket Costs under Medicare.* Washington, DC: U.S. Congressional Budget Office.

———. 1988. *The Medicare Catastrophic Coverage Act of 1988.* Washington, DC: U.S. Congressional Budget Office.

———. 1989a. *A Background Material on the Catastrophic Drug Insurance Program.* Washington, DC: U.S. Congressional Budget Office.

———. 1989b. *The Economic Status of the Elderly.* Washington, DC: U.S. Congressional Budget Office.

———. 1991. *Universal Health Insurance Coverage Using Medicare's Payment Rates.* Washington, DC: U.S. Government Printing Office.

———. 2002. *Budget Options*. Washington, DC: U.S. Government Printing Office.

———. 2003. *The Budget and Economic Outlook: Fiscal Years 2004–2013*. Washington, DC: U.S. Congressional Budget Office.

———. 2004. *A Detailed Description of CBO's Cost Estimate for the Medicare Prescription Drug Benefit*. Washington, DC: U.S. Congressional Budget Office.

———. 2005. *Budget Options*. Washington, DC: U.S. Congressional Budget Office.

U.S. Department of Health and Human Services. 1986. *Catastrophic Illness Expenses*. Report to the President. Washington, DC: U.S. Department of Health and Human Services.

———. 2001. *Health Care Financing Review: Medicare and Medicaid Statistical Supplement, 2000*. Baltimore, MD: Centers for Medicare and Medicaid Services.

———. 2003. *2003 CMS Statistics*. Baltimore, MD: Centers for Medicare and Medicaid Services.

U.S. General Accounting Office. 1998. *Medigap Insurance: Compliance with Federal Standards Has Increased*. Washington, DC: U.S. General Accounting Office.

———. 2000. "Medicare + Choice: Payments Exceed Cost of Fee-for-Service Benefits, Adding Billions to Spending." Report no. GAO/HEHS-00-161. Washington, DC: U.S. General Accounting Office.

———. 2001. "Medicare + Choice: Recent Payment Increases Had Little Effect on Benefits or Plan Availability in 2001." Report no. GAO-02-202. Washington, DC: U.S. General Accounting Office.

———. 2002. *Long-Term Care: Aging Baby Boom Generation Will Increase Demand and Burden on Federal and State Budgets*. Washington, DC: U.S. General Accounting Office.

U.S. Government Accountability Office. 2004. "Medicare Demonstration PPOs: Financial and Other Advantages for Plans, Few Advantages for Beneficiaries." Report no. GAO-04-960. Washington, DC: U.S. Government Accountability Office.

U.S. Social Security Administration. 1991. *Annual Statistical Supplement to the Social Security Bulletin, 1991*. Washington, DC: U.S. Government Printing Office.

Waidmann, Timothy. 1998. "Potential Effects of Raising Medicare's Eligibility Age." *Health Affairs* 17 (March/April): 156–64.

Waldo, Daniel, Sally Sonnefeld, David McKusick, and Ross Arnett. 1989. "Health Expenditures by Age Group, 1977 and 1987." *Health Care Financing Review* 10 (Summer): 111–20.

Webster's. 1966. *New World Dictionary of the American Language*. Cleveland: The World Publishing Co.

Weiss, Linda, and Jan Blustein. 1996. "Faithful Patients: The Effect of Long-Term Physician-Patient Relationships on the Costs and Use of Health Care by Older Americans." *American Journal of Public Health* 86 (December): 1742–47.

Weiss Ratings, Inc. 2003. "Consumers Face Huge Disparities in Medigap Rates." July 14. http://www.weissratings.com/News/Ins_Medigap.

Wiener, Joshua M., Lauren Illston, and Raymond Hanley. 1994. *Sharing the Burden: Strategies for Public and Private Long-Term Care Insurance*. Washington, DC: The Brookings Institution.

ABOUT THE AUTHOR

M arilyn Moon is vice president and director of the Health Program at the American Institutes for Research. A nationally known expert on Medicare, she has served as a senior fellow at the Urban Institute and as a public trustee for the Social Security and Medicare trust funds. Dr. Moon has written extensively on health policy, both for the elderly and the population in general, and on social insurance issues. From 1993 to 2000, Moon also wrote a periodic column for the *Washington Post* on health reform and health coverage issues. She has served on a number of boards for nonprofit organizations and is currently president of the board of the Medicare Rights Center and the National Academy of Social Insurance. She is a member of the Institute of Medicine of the National Academy of Sciences. Previously, she has been an associate professor of economics at the University of Wisconsin–Milwaukee, a senior analyst at the Congressional Budget Office, and the founding director of the Public Policy Institute of the American Association of Retired Persons.

INDEX